The Love-Your-Heart Guide for the 1990s

LEE BELSHIN, M.S.

Good Health
Lee Belshin

CB
CONTEMPORARY
BOOKS
CHICAGO

Library of Congress Cataloging-in-Publication Data

Belshin, Leon.
  The love-your-heart guide for the 1990s : the most up-
to-date information for complete heart health / Lee Belshin.
      p.   cm.
  Includes index.
  ISBN 0-8092-4096-3 (paper) : $7.95
      1. Heart—Infarction—Prevention.   2. Self-care, Health.
  I. Title.
  RC685.I6B44   1990
  616.1'205—dc20   90-42279
                                                          CIP

Grateful acknowledgment is made for permission to use material from the following:

"The Coronary Club" from "Managing Your Stress" by Dr. Martin E. Keller. Reprinted with permission from Life Association News; Volume 81, No. 12 (December 1986).

"Drugs Used in Treating High Blood Pressure" reprinted by permission from Coffey Communications, Inc.

"the shoelace" copyright 1972 by Charles Bukowski. Reprinted from *Mockingbird Wish Me Luck* with the permission of Black Sparrow Press.

"Vulnerability Scale" from the *Stress Audit*, developed by Lyle H. Miller and Alma Dell Smith. Copyright 1983, Biobehavioral Associates, Brookline, MA 02146. Reprinted with permission.

To Joan Belshin, a career counselor, who has helped so many people to rediscover themselves as she has helped me for 40 years of our marriage; and to my daughter, Maryann; and sons, Joseph and Matthew, constant sources of inspiration

Contents

Foreword

It is most unusual for someone who is working in the insurance and financial field to be active in coronary prevention programs. But such is the case with Lee Belshin. His experience as a health educator and teacher of gerontology has given him considerable insight into the need for educating the public about how to prevent coronary artery disease.

I first became associated with Lee Belshin while he was serving as president of the American Heart Association, Northern California Golden Empire Chapter. From that a relationship developed that resulted in the book *Love Your Heart*.

His new book, *The Love-Your-Heart Guide for the 1990s*, is an updated version that provides the reader with the latest research on how to prevent a fatal heart attack. Most important, it is scientifically sound, yet written in a style that is easy for the reader to understand so he or she can immediately apply this vital knowledge.

In addition to serving as editor in chief of the *American Heart Journal*, I have authored more than 1,000 original articles for professional journals and 10 textbooks on several aspects of cardiovascular science and clinical cardiology. So I am well aware of the importance of a book such as this, which provides advice on how to protect yourself and your family from the leading cause of death.

Dean T. Mason, M.D.
Physician in Chief,
Western Heart Institute
Chairman, Department of
Cardiovascular Medicine
St. Mary's Medical Center
San Francisco, California

Acknowledgments

This book has been made possible by the support and encouragement of many individuals in the medical profession and related fields. The support of physicians, especially in the western states, was essential in gathering the lifesaving information presented in this book.

I would like to give special thanks to Dr. Edward B. Johns, professor emeritus of the UCLA School of Public Health, who has given me the background and motivation to write this book.

The information provided by John Yudkin, M.D., of London; Mrs. Phillip Gillon of the Hadassah-Hebrew University Medical Center in Israel; and other health officials throughout the world was extremely helpful. I also want to thank David Morgan for his literary assistance.

Introduction

The research required to write this book was truly a labor of love. It involved talking to many people both in and out of the medical profession. I wrote my first book on preventing cardiac disease, and now this one, because I have seen so much needless loss of life. So many of my friends in the insurance and the financial planning professions have died in the prime of life from a sudden heart attack.

My father died of a heart attack at the age of 59 at my wedding. It was a period of his life when he should have been enjoying the fruits of his labor. That experience certainly demonstrated to me what a tremendous impact sudden death has on a family.

But my lifesaving mission really started one day while I was seated on a plane returning from a sales conference. I glanced at an open page of the *Million Dollar Round Table* magazine. In it was an article entitled "In Memory Of." The names were well known to me: young family men about my age, all leaders in their respective companies. Once again a fatal heart attack was the villain that brought all of their promising careers to a sudden end.

When I returned to Sacramento, I attended several funerals of other salespersons in my age group. The oldest was 46; he left six young children and a wife to

face the future without support. That did it. I stormed
into the local Heart Association office and asked, "Can
you use me? I am a former public health educator with a
master of science degree in health education from
UCLA and considerable speaking experience."

"You bet we can," they responded.

I then became chairperson of the speaker's bureau of
the Golden Empire Council of the American Heart Association. Immediately I began to talk to many groups
about preventing coronary heart disease.

Was there a need? Absolutely.

Requests piled in, and every time I spoke the audience
asked hundreds of questions about avoiding heart disease. As a result I began to devote more and more time
to the Heart Association and eventually became president of the Golden Empire Chapter and received their
distinguished service award.

My greatest rewards, however, came after each talk.
At least one person would come up and say, "Lee, you
really got me. I am going to quit smoking and start on a
regular exercise program. I wish I had heard you last
year. I just had a bypass operation, and my physician
said I should do exactly what you have now recommended."

Then letters began to pour in from all over the country from salespersons and others pleading for information that could help save their lives. I had a real message
to get across. Yet one day, while seated in an airport
waiting for my plane, I realized that with all my good
intentions I was barely scratching the surface.

So my first book, *Love Your Heart*, was born. I was
most fortunate that Dean T. Mason, M.D., one of the
most prominent cardiologists in the United States and
editor of the *American Heart Journal*, also realized the
need for a book based on scientific knowledge. He helped
me by carefully reviewing the book to make sure the

content was accurate and current. He presented the book to William B. Kannel, M.D., a well-known epidemiologist and former director of the famous Framingham study. After reading it, Dr. Kannel agreed to write the foreword.

The book received considerable support from the medical community. It was approved for cardiac nurses' training in several states and is used by colleges as a text for health education classes. All of this increased my speaking load.

The original *Love Your Heart* was written in the early 1980s. Since that time a great deal of research has added significantly to our knowledge about how cardiac disease develops and how to prevent it. For this reason I have written its sequel for the next decade, *The Love-Your-Heart Guide for the 1990s.*

This book is dedicated to executives, salespersons, engineers, teachers, retirees, homemakers, and every other American who wants to live a long, healthy life free of cardiac health problems. It will show you how to bypass a bypass. More than 350,000 Americans have bypass surgery a year, a very high number for a procedure that many physicians find controversial.

Essentially, this book is a formula to help you live longer, enhance your enjoyment of life, and increase your productivity.

One of the problems I found when I started talking to people was their belief that they couldn't continue their present robust lifestyle and still carry out a complete cardiac prevention program.

A senior vice president of one of the companies that I represent, who was familiar with my work, said, "Lee, I know you are on a 26-state tour to show salespeople how to increase productivity. That's a pretty hectic schedule. I bet even you will add at least 20 pounds. You will be eating in restaurants and will most likely not have time

to continue your daily exercise program." I should have
accepted the wager, for he was wrong. In fact, I lost two
pounds.

I was highly motivated to continue my morning exercise program. Anytime I felt like abstaining for a day I
could hear Dr. David B. Rutstein of the Harvard Medical School whispering in my ear, "Since the heart is
chiefly a muscle, exercise makes it extremely tough."
And although I don't go back that far, I could hear
Hippocrates in 400 B.C. admonishing his patients, "That
which is used develops; that which is not deteriorates." If
I still felt like lying in bed I could picture Dr. Joseph B.
Wolfe, head of the Valley Forge Heart Hospital, shouting
at me, "Lee Belshin, it is important to note that the
heart gains strength through work which produces extra blood supply with better nourishment. Regular exercise with periods of rest is the most important measure
against disease of the heart."

In the end, I always got out of bed raring to go—well,
if not raring, at least motivated.

And that's really the reason I wrote this book. With it
I want to motivate you to control those lifestyle factors
that threaten your heart health.

Now, it's up to you. Your life is in your hands. It is my
wish that you hear the message in this book, make the
few lifestyle changes needed, and survive to a very old
age. And when you do, I hope you will hear my voice in
your ear saying, "I told you you could do it . . . now have
a very healthy life."

1
Whole Heart Health

Last year almost a million men and women in the United States—many of them in the prime of life—died of heart disease. This year an even greater number will die. Heart attacks kill one out of every four people in the nation, more than all other causes of death combined. A life is taken every 32 seconds. In a single year diseases of the heart and blood vessels kill more Americans than died in World Wars I and II, and the Korean and Vietnam wars.

The saddest thing about this is that most of these unfortunate victims did not have to die. If they had just taken the few simple precautions that will be outlined in this book, they would probably still be around today. What a waste! What a tragic loss to their families. What a tremendous loss to the country.

Unfortunately, many of you who are now reading this book are candidates for a heart attack this year. Even worse, you could have had one or more heart attacks during the past year without even knowing it. Impossible? Not as impossible as you might think. Doctors conducting autopsies are often amazed at the many scars in the heart muscle caused by heart attacks too mild to be recognized. What's more, you may now be walking around with a time bomb that could go off any moment. And repeated attacks, no matter how mild, will eventually lead to a fatal attack unless you start to take preventive steps right now.

One tragic death, several years ago, convinced me to write my first book, *Love Your Heart*. I had an appointment with a 44-year-old former army officer who was married and had three children. Having just purchased a new home, he wanted to discuss increasing his life insurance to protect his family. I arrived early and waited on the couch while they finished dinner.

He was overweight and was consuming an enormous meal high in saturated fat: a salad topped with rich dressing, meat smothered in gravy, potatoes with butter, and apple pie and ice cream. He finished dinner and walked over to where I was seated. He was breathing hard from this exertion, and his face was flushed. Obviously he was in poor condition. I could contain myself no longer.

"You hardly know me," I said, "and you may very well throw me out of your home, but I want to talk about your health. You just finished a dinner loaded with cholesterol, you're overweight, you smoke, and you're huffing and puffing from a walk to the couch. You're a prime candidate for a heart attack." At this point his wife shouted out, "Give it to him. I've been telling him that for years."

My client, however, did not want to discuss his health any further, so I sold him the life insurance policy he wanted. He was confident that he would pass the physical since he had just passed his army discharge exam with flying colors. However, the insurance physician discovered he had high blood pressure. This meant he would pay a higher premium.

When I delivered the policy, I recommended that he place himself under a doctor's care to reduce his weight, learn to eat a healthy diet, and bring down the blood pressure. Unfortunately he refused to take my advice.

The next month, he dropped dead from a heart attack,

leaving behind a young widow and three children. This death could have been prevented, because the conditions that led to his death had been building up for a long time.

It is tragedies such as this that led me to write the first book on preventing heart attacks, and now this one, *The Love-Your-Heart Guide for the 1990s.* My entire purpose—if you are at risk—is to motivate you to take immediate steps to reduce the risk factors for coronary disease that may exist in your present lifestyle. Or, if you have already experienced a heart attack and survived, to make sure you never experience another. Now, together, let's start the journey toward good heart health.

CORONARY DISEASE RISKS

You should be aware of a number of factors that will increase your risk of coronary disease. In this chapter we will survey them briefly. In the remaining chapters you will learn the many ways to reduce and control each one. Here are the factors to consider. Controllable factors are lack of exercise, high blood pressure, cholesterol levels, obesity, elevated blood sugar, other diet factors, smoking, alcohol, and stress. Uncontrollable factors are age, race, family history, and sex. Let's quickly look at the major ones.

Exercise

Almost everyone today knows that exercise is an important factor in preventing cardiac disease, yet very few realize how significant it really is. In the 1950s a still-quoted British Research Council study conducted by Dr. J. N. Morris, which surveyed the records of 5,000 men who died in British hospitals, discovered that those who had been in physically active jobs had a significantly lower incidence of coronary heart disease than those in sedentary jobs, and Dr. Morris's more recent studies have supported this. The original study also revealed that London bus drivers who sat down all day had a much higher rate of heart disease than the conductors who walked up and down.

An Israeli study of 9,000 inhabitants of 58 communal settlements found that over half of the coronary disease cases were in the inactive group, and the death rate of sedentary workers was three to four times that of active workers. Prompted by a lack of solid findings in previous research on physical activity and heart disease, the United States Centers for Disease Control recently launched a two-year analysis of 43 previous studies of cardiac heart disease and exercise. The overall review concluded that lack of exercise may be as strongly linked to heart disease as smoking, high blood pressure, and high cholesterol.

Currently many authorities—such as the late Dr. Paul Dudley White; Dr. Terence Kavanagh, director of the Toronto Cardiac Rehabilitation Centre; William Kannel, M.D., medical director of the Framingham, Mass., study; Dr. Jean Mayer, president of Tufts Medical College; and Dr. Kenneth Cooper—are militant in their support of regular lifelong exercise. Chapter 2 will help match your lifestyle to exercise or exercises that work best for you.

High Blood Pressure

High blood pressure is called the "silent killer" because it has no symptoms as it sets up its victims for heart attacks, strokes, and other disabling diseases. More than 60 million Americans today have high blood pressure. And as many as two-thirds either have not been diagnosed or are not being adequately treated, which means that more than 40 million people who desperately need treatment are simply not getting it. In Chapter 4 you will find a number of tips for controlling blood pressure and methods to help reduce this threat.

Nutrition

Despite the current interest in health and nutrition, the average individual's diet still leaves a lot to be desired. A study by the U.S. Department of Agriculture showed that 21 percent of Americans were getting less than two-thirds of the necessary nutrients. In a later study by the same group, adolescents between 10 and 16 had the worst diet, while the diets of elderly Americans were deficient in at least two of the food groups.

A 1976 study among epidemiologists, nutritionists, geneticists, and other research scientists showed that 92 percent believed there was a relationship between diet and heart disease significant enough to recommend a reduction in the number of calories and fat consumed. In addition, a more recent study by the National Cancer Institute concluded that most Americans were still ignoring diet as a contributing factor to both heart disease and cancer. The American diet is very poor, and people are dying because of it.

According to nutrition expert and government consultant Dr. Theodore Van Sittalie, "There is a strong link between obesity and heart disease, but it is not entirely clear whether this is because obese people are often more sedentary and have a tendency toward diabetes, hypertension, and other problems." Says Dr. Joseph B. Herman of the Hadassah-Hebrew University Medical Center, Jerusalem, "Since diseases of the blood vessels, including coronary heart disease in particular, have been known for years to be related to diabetes, it should make us more determined to keep weight down." Unfortunately a recent study has shown that more Americans are more overweight than ever before, and the *American Journal of Diseases of Children* reports that obesity has increased 54 percent in children between 6 and 11, and 39 percent in adolescents and teenagers between 12 and 17.

There are other nutritional factors. Nutritionist Dr.

John Yudkin feels strongly that sugar may be just as injurious to heart health as animal fat or cholesterol. Chapter 3 gives you the information you need to eat in a healthy way and reduce the probability of your diet contributing to coronary disease.

Smoking

Smoking causes an estimated 390,000 heart disease-related deaths each year. Many studies, including the famous 40-year Framingham heart study, conducted on 5,000 Massachusetts volunteers free from heart disease to determine the dangers of blood cholesterol, have found that protective HDL levels are lower for men and women who smoke. HDL (high-density lipoprotein) cholesterol transports cholesterol for removal from the body and is thus called the "good" cholesterol. Generally, the higher a person's HDL level, the better. It has also been shown that secondhand smoking creates many heart health problems for nonsmokers, especially pregnant women. A recent joint study by the University of California and the University of Utah of 7,000 smokers indicates that nonsmoking wives of smokers are 3.4 times more vulnerable to heart attacks than are wives of men who don't smoke. Explains Dr. William Moskowitz of the Virginia Medical College, "Our preliminary findings also indicate that cigarette smoke affects the heart and blood fat of 12-year-old boys severely and may put them at even higher risk in the following decades."

The battery of poisons and pollutants contained in cigarette smoke also causes numerous heart-related problems. Kyoto University research showed that cigarette smoke modifies LDL in the bloodstream, causing it to lay down increased artery-clogging plaque. LDL (low-density lipoprotein) cholesterol collects cholesterol and deposits it in our cells and is thus known as "bad" cholesterol. Chapter 5 explains the problem and offers several methods to kick the smoking habit.

Alcohol

According to Dr. Marvin Moser, clinical professor of medicine at the New York Medical College and the senior medical consultant to the National High Blood Pressure Education program of the National Heart, Lung, and Blood Institute, besides alcohol's devastating effect on the liver and brain, "there is also some evidence that heavy use of alcohol—more than 4-5 drinks a day—can raise blood pressure." And although it has been suggested that the alcohol in an occasional drink or two may help raise HDL (the "good" cholesterol) levels, the vote is not in yet on whether alcohol's negative effects outweigh that possible benefit.

Stress

Stress disorders cost industry an estimated $17 to $25 million annually. Stress itself causes headaches, high blood pressure, alcoholism, ulcers, suicides, and heart attacks. How stress affects each individual, according to Meyer Friedman, M.D., depends on whether he or she is Type A or Type B. Recent research, however, has shown that personality type may not be as important in predicting heart attacks as how that person handles the stress he or she encounters.

Chapter 6 explains the stress/distress concept, offers self-diagnostic stress symptoms, and includes a test to help determine personality type.

WHAT'S YOUR CARDIAC RISK?

A portrait of the prime candidate for cardiac disease in the 1990s is a middle-aged man or elderly female who craves rich, fatty foods, smokes cigarettes, refuses to exercise, and reacts to stress with anger and hostility.

Unfortunately, research shows that cardiac disease is not confined to this group but extends almost from birth to death for both males and females. Let's look at some of the individual groups and see just what your risk is.

Male Children, 12 and Under

Can children really have symptoms of heart disease? They not only can, but they also have a more serious problem than first realized. A University of California at Davis study of 95 boys aged 8 to 12 showed that many had the same risk factors heart specialists find in middle-aged patients. A similar study in Ann Arbor, Michigan, found that nearly half of a group of 400 children showed risk factors including abnormally high cholesterol levels, high blood pressure, and obesity. Say Drs. Robert Voller and William Strong, writing in the *American Heart Journal*, "Atherosclerosis and coronary heart disease continue to be major health problems in the United States and other industrialized nations." Atherosclerosis, a form of arteriosclerosis (commonly called hardening of the arteries), causes the artery walls to become thick and irregular from deposits, called plaque, of cholesterol and other substances. The arteries are narrower, which reduces the flow of blood. Although these manifestations usually do not appear until adult life, they apparently have their origins in childhood.

It follows then that parents must start preventive measures at an early age, especially for boys. This means watching the consumption of doughnuts, potato chips, hamburgers, and soda pop and substituting the balanced foods offered in Chapter 3.

Male Teenagers

If the problems that trigger coronary disease actually start in early childhood, it stands to reason that teenagers would exhibit even more severe symptoms.

Autopsies performed during the Korean War on 300 American soldiers, ranging in age from teens to early twenties, showed that 77 percent had evidence of hardening of the coronary arteries and blood clots that had already damaged their hearts. During the Vietnam War, 45 percent of the casualties examined had signs of coronary disease before their deaths. One out of ten had his coronary arteries blocked more than 50 percent, and 1 in 4 had a blockage of 20 percent. The conclusion was that even if these soldiers had survived the war and returned to their former lifestyles, they would have been prime candidates for an early heart attack.

Some nutritionists now feel that teenagers especially should watch their diets and their cholesterol levels. This means limiting hamburgers, french fries, milk shakes, packaged foods, and other high-fat-content items such as mayonnaise, butter, and margarine and adding chicken, fish, legumes, whole-wheat grain products, and vegetables.

Males in their Twenties, Thirties, and Forties
A study of more than 200 pilots, average age 28, killed in plane crashes during World War II showed that 6 percent had severe blockage of the coronary arteries, while 2 percent had already had a heart attack. Dr. Paul Dudley White, commenting on autopsies that he and his associates had performed on 350 Boston heart attack victims, stated that they failed to find a clean artery in any person over 21 years old. And although these studies were done several years ago, they show the permanent damage that can be done in youth. Medically speaking, middle age now begins in a man's twenties. And Dr. Ancel Keys adds, "Among adults in the United States, the question is not who has atherosclerosis, but rather who has more and who has less."

The typical American in the 20 through 50 age group now consumes 75 pounds of beef a year, 44 pounds of pork, 40 pounds of chicken, 40 gallons of soda, and 110 pounds of sugar. Reports former Surgeon General C. Everett Koop, "They, like most other groups of Americans, need desperately to cut down on the amount of saturated fats in their diets." Researchers have also found that this group tends to be much too sedentary, spending an inordinate amount of time either in the car or in front of the television set. Most would do well to also devote at least 30 minutes a day three times a week to performing some type of aerobic exercise. A recent study performed on 3,106 healthy men aged 30–59 demonstrated that regular endurance training may well be effective in preventing coronary heart disease and in promoting general good health for this age group.

Males over 55

Among men over 55, researchers find that many of the physical symptoms of aging are merely the result of inactivity. Their findings also indicate that even moderate exercise can retard the effects of aging and even reverse them. The important thing at this age is to keep moving. Sports fitness experts say that walking is a perfect exercise after 50. But they also recommend joining seniors' fitness programs that include swimming and other forms of aerobics. Nutrition is also critical for seniors. It is important at this age, studies show, to maintain a healthy diet, keep fat intake to a minimum, and lower the cholesterol level.

Women

Contrary to popular belief, coronary heart disease is not uncommon in women. Of the more than 520,000 fatal heart attacks that occur every year, 247,000 of them strike women.

Women in their thirties and forties appear to have a built-in immunity to heart disease as long as they menstruate. Estrogen, a female hormone produced by menstruating women, increases the level of "good" cholesterol. When women reach menopause, their risk of developing heart disease increases. If menopause occurs naturally, the risk develops more slowly. If menopause is caused by hysterectomy, the risk rises sharply. But just because a woman is still ovulating does not mean she is immune to heart attack.

One in 9 women between the ages of 45 and 64 has

some form of cardiovascular disease; the ratio for women over 65 is 1 in 8. In addition, 56 percent of women with heart disease will become aware of it due to angina pectoris, or chest pain. Often this symptom will go undiagnosed for years because a woman is less likely than a man to wonder if the pain is heart related. Women are twice as likely to die within the first two weeks after a heart attack as men, and 39 percent die within the first year. In addition stroke kills over 90,000 women each year within this age group.

All of this means that postmenopausal women should become as heart-conscious as men and watch their cholesterol, exercise regularly, and get a treadmill stress test to determine any initial signs of heart problems.

Finally, during the 1970s, a strong connection was made between diet and the increased tendency toward atherosclerosis and heart disease in diabetics. Now it is recommended that diabetics follow the standard techniques for preventing cardiac disease. Health agencies now feel that it is also crucial for diabetics to add more fiber to their diets, since fiber seems to help stabilize fluctuating blood sugar levels.

No matter who you are, however, man or woman, young or old, the remaining chapters of this book will help you put together an individualized comprehensive program that will help decrease your overall risk of coronary heart disease.

HEART ATTACK SYMPTOMS

Should you have a heart attack, however, it is important to know and be able to recognize the signs. The symptoms can come on gradually or occur without any apparent warning even in people who never before experienced any chest pain. The important thing is not to deny or ignore your pain. The earlier you get help, the less chance of permanent disability or death, especially now that there are better-than-ever treatments waiting to assist you.

The Warning Signals

• Uncomfortable pressure, fullness, squeezing, or pain in the center of the chest lasting two minutes or longer

• Pain spreading to the back, shoulders, neck, jaw, or arms

• Sweating, nausea, dizziness, panting, shortness of breath, or weakness

Not every heart-attack victim experiences every symptom. The American Heart Association advises you to call an ambulance or have someone quickly drive you to the hospital if your pain lasts two minutes or more.

2
Exercise for Your
Heart's Sake

Better to hunt in fields, for health unbought,
Than fee the doctor for a nauseous draught,
The wise, for cure, on exercise depend;
God never made his work, for man to mend.

—John Dryden's 17th-century beliefs

When you think about it, the heart is truly an amazing organ. It begins to beat months before you are born and continues to beat at least once every second, every day, every year of your life, propelling oxygen and other nutrients to every one of the many billions of cells in the body through a blood-vessel network whose length is more than four times the circumference of the earth.

Your heart is an untiring organ, beating about 100,000 times daily, 40 million times a year. Unlike a clock, the heart, with only a fraction of a second's rest between beats, does not need rewinding. It continues to pump for a lifetime. That lifetime depends, to a great extent, on how we treat this vital organ. This tiny organ, about the size of a clenched fist, moves more than 4,000 gallons, or 10 tons, of blood each day and every night—a task equivalent to carrying a 30-pound pack to the top of the Empire State Building. Is it too much to ask that we give our heart enough exercise to keep it fit and us alive? The answer is, of course not!

THE EXERCISE EFFECT

Exercise is currently considered an essential tool for anyone on a cardiac disease prevention program. Numerous research studies now provide evidence that exercise strengthens the heart. Drs. J. Naughton and J. Brughn of the Division of Cardiology, George Washington University, report that men who do not exercise have twice as many heart attacks as those who are physically active; they suggest that if suitable exercise programs are started early in life, these heart attacks should be preventable. Drs. S. M. Fox III, J. Naughton, and W. L. Haskell found evidence that increased exercise can definitely help prevent heart disease.

Dr. Wilhelm Raabb of the University of Vermont College of Medicine, serving on an international team of scientists studying the problem of heart disease, pointed out that lack of exercise is a serious threat to Western civilization. "It is not the so-called athlete's heart which should be considered abnormal," he says, "but rather the degenerating, inadequate loafer's heart."

Dr. Joan Ullyot, director of the Institute of Health Research, San Francisco, states, "Instead of concentration on cures, the medical professional should spend a lot more time on prevention, and one of the best ways to prevent a lot of disorders of modern society is by regular, vigorous exercise—and I mean vigorous in terms of what it does for the heart and lungs."

Runner Clarence Demar offers a good example of what exercise can do. While a student at the University of Vermont, he was a cross-country runner with great potential. After he won the Boston Marathon, however, his doctors told him he had a weak heart and should stop running. He ignored this advice and competed in more than 1,000 long-distance races, including 100 marathons of 25 miles or more. He also ran the Boston Marathon 34 times and won this grueling race 7 times. His last race, a year before his death at age 70 from cancer, was a 10-mile one. When internationally known cardiologist Dr. Paul Dudley White examined his heart, he found it contained two coronary arteries that were two to three times normal size. Although Demar's heart artery was narrowed by as much as 30 percent in several spots, there was still plenty of room, because of the artery's size, to allow a more than adequate flow of blood to the heart. Dr. James Currens, former assistant in medicine, Massachusetts General Hospital, who also studied Demar's heart, concluded that "when you exercise or work hard physically, your heart muscle must work harder and more efficiently to distribute blood to all parts of the body, including its own muscular tissue. A more extensive network of blood channels (known as collateral circulation) develops to ensure a good supply of blood." This development apparently is what gave Demar a long and active life.

New research shows that physiologically the body undergoes an adaptive response to the demands of repeated aerobic exercise. The heart grows larger and expels more blood with each beat, inducing increased capillary formation. The lung capacity increases, and the exercised muscles become more efficient and develop higher concentrations of energy-generating enzymes. This is called the "training effect."

OTHER BENEFITS

Besides a direct effect on the heart, exercise has an indirect effect on some of the other risk factors. Reports Dr. Peter D. Wood, "Exercise is a kind of an all purpose risk reducer. It not only improves cardiovascular efficiency but helps reduce stress, bring down high blood pressure, and control obesity."

Says Dr. Kenneth Cooper, founder of the Aerobics Center in Dallas, Texas (considered to be responsible for the exercise boom sweeping the country), "Real physical exercise erases mental fatigue." The first systematic study of the effects of exercise on the nervous system was conducted in 1953 by Dr. Thomas Cureton, professor of physical education, University of Illinois. Studying 2,500 adults over a 10-year period, Dr. Cureton became convinced that physical exercise helps alleviate nervous tension.

Studies now show that tense people have tight, contracted muscles with high levels of electrical activity. Dr. Herbert DeVries, an exercise physiologist at the University of Southern California, found that the electrical activity in the muscles of a group of college teachers dropped 255 percent after five weeks of exercise.

Many people who exercise regularly recognize this benefit. I work in a highly competitive industry but find that as long as I exercise I can cope. Several years ago after I mentioned this in a Rotary Club talk, a stockbroker called to thank me. He was convinced that exercise had reduced his risk of coronary disease and changed his entire lifestyle. The pressures of his job had left him so tense at the end of the day that he would go home feeling nervous and angry. He now parks his car blocks away and briskly walks to and from the office. During the long walk, he says, he can feel the stress in his mind and body disappear.

Exercise also helps reduce obesity—a heart attack risk. Student health services director Dr. C. Herman Brown has shown that regular exercise changes fat into lean muscle and allows you to sleep more deeply and awaken feeling refreshed at the end of the night. University of Pennsylvania psychologist Kelly P. Beowell reports that if people would walk up and down a mere two floors of stairs a day, instead of taking the elevator, they could lose six pounds or more over the course of a year.

Many gerontologists also feel that exercise helps keep

the heart in shape to a very advanced age. Dr. Wildor Hollman, professor of sports medicine and cardiology at the Cologne University Institute for Sports Medicine, reported that while physical activity does not counter the development of arteriosclerosis with advancing age, it helps the capillary network to supplement the blood supply to such vital areas as the heart muscle.

Studies show that senior citizens who exercise regularly do not show the typical symptoms of aging, such as slowed reflex times, reduced muscle tone, and bone brittleness. Indeed many now claim that they feel more fit than they did when they were much younger and less physically active.

Larry Lewis, the star of the film *Run Dick, Run Jane*, was found at his death to have a strong, healthy heart. Lewis ran consistently for 94 years and was still running a few years before his death at 106. Harvard nonagenarian Dean Roscoe Pound walked thousands of miles through Scotland, Ireland, and France at an advanced age. And feisty Harry Truman, who lived to be 88, often complained that he had to slow his walking pace for the much younger reporters. Rose Kennedy walked four to five miles every day until her ninetieth birthday. When I carried mail during the cold winter days in Boston, I used to marvel at the elderly carriers who would trek through the streets and up and down the stairs all day. They all looked so hardy and robust.

Fortunately, more and more seniors are beginning to take part in some form of exercise. For instance, of the 18,000 runners in a recent New York Marathon, 4,719 were in their fifties, 217 were in their sixties, 19 were over 70, and 1 was 80 plus. Other types of exercise now attract millions of participants who are in their nineties and beyond.

In a 1987 Finnish study first published in the British medical journal *Lancet*, the activities and physical characteristics of 635 Finnish males aged 45 to 64 were followed for up to 20 years. After adjustments were made for age, smoking, weight gain, blood pressure, and serum cholesterol levels, it became clear that vigorous and regular physical activity such as long-distance walking, bicycling, and cross-country skiing could add at least two additional years to a person's life.

To test this theory, USC researchers are now comparing the physical changes that occur in nonathletes with those that are experienced by the so-called Master Athletes, people over 40 who continue, despite their age, to compete in sports. Among the 200 to 300 older athletes, Robert A. Wiswell, an associate professor in USC's Department of Physical Education and Exercise Sciences, hopes to monitor over the next 20 years are a woman who took up long-distance running in middle age, a 75-year-old man who holds the world record in pole vaulting for his age group, and an 87-year-old who runs at least 90 5- to 10-kilometer races a year. Although it will be years before the final results of the USC study are known, many researchers are already beginning to draw conclusions. USC professor of gerontology Ruth Wig is uncomfortable, as are many health experts, with the idea of waiting until all the data is in to start changing lifestyles and reforming eating habits. "We may not have all the answers we need," she says, "but we know enough now to at least start." Her prescription is simple: begin moderate exercise immediately and do it regularly, then add a diet neither too high in calories nor too rich in cholesterol.

Recent studies in physiology also show that properly prescribed exercise in middle to old age can actually turn back the clock physiologically 10 to 25 years. Dr. Roy J. Shephard, an expert on exercise and aging from the University of Toronto, summed it up by saying, "It now appears, after all, that exercise may well turn out to be the long elusive fountain of youth."

In 1968, Herbert A. DeVries, then one of the country's few experts in the field of exercise and aging, predicted that the time will come when it will be possible to prescribe exercise for an individual with the same scientific detail and exactness as that now employed in writing a prescription for medicines. Gerontologists, who specialize in the science of aging, are very optimistic that in a few years they may well be able to disrupt the aging process through proper use of exercise so that many people in their eighties and nineties will be as physically fit and mentally alert as any 50-year-old. Researchers have also found that exercise coupled with a restricted caloric intake has successfully doubled the life span of laboratory rodents.

Hippocrates, the ancient Greek physician, stated in 400 B.C., "Speaking generally, all parts of the body which have a function, if used in moderation and exercised in labors in which each is accustomed, thereby become healthy, well developed, and age more slowly, but if bruised and left idle they become liable to disease, defective in growth, and age more quickly."

THE VITAL CHECK-UP

Before you actually start any exercise program, you should get a physical exam. This will alert you to any physical problems that might be exacerbated through exercise and need to be corrected before continuing. For instance, starting on a program when you have undetected high blood pressure could put an immediate end to your program and even your life.

The exam should include an electrocardiogram (EKG), administered during exercise, that pinpoints areas around the heart where oxygen supplies are low.

This way, about 80 percent of all individuals with coronary blockage can be screened. The American College of Sports Medicine suggests that this test be required for all individuals over 35 years of age. It should also be required for anyone under 35 who has a high risk of heart disease and is recommended for all others. During this test you will be wired to an EKG machine and made to breathe into a metabolic computer as you walk on a treadmill whose speed and grade are increased on the minute. While the EKG scope blips out the rhythm of your heart, you run to the point of voluntary exhaustion to see how your heart functions under extreme stress.

The ability of your heart to tolerate stress is one of the key factors to be considered in prescribing an exercise program tailored to your individual needs and limitations. As Dr. John Davis Cantwell says, "A doctor can't make a complete assessment of the heart in its resting state any more than a professional coach can assess the capability of a rookie quarterback by merely observing him on the bench. The heart, like the quarterback, must be observed in action."

In addition to an EKG, a thorough physical examination will include an analysis of a blood sample to determine your cholesterol level. Cholesterol is the tasteless, odorless, white, fatty alcohol found in oils and in all animal fats. Lipoprotein and triglyceride levels should also be measured. Lipoproteins are the fat-protein combinations found in the blood. Triglycerides are not cholesterol but fatty molecules in your blood. They are considered by many heart specialists to be as risky as cholesterol.

WHAT KIND OF EXERCISE?

Research shows that any exercise that benefits the heart and helps prevent cardiac disease must be aerobic. That is, it must be strenuous enough to increase the efficiency of the oxygen intake to the heart and lungs and help build the heart muscle and condition the arteries. Dr. Kenneth Cooper, while conducting studies in the U.S. Air Force, discovered that aerobic exercise must be consistent over a period of time and must increase the heart rate to the point where you can obtain "training effect" benefits. The standard today is at least three 20-minute aerobic sessions a week.

The American College of Sports Medicine recommends that you establish a safe training zone for effective exercise pulse rates based on your age and level of fitness and that you calculate both 70 percent and 85 percent of your maximum heart rate to find the low and high ends of your range. Here's how to do it.

To determine your target zone for optimal performance (for men), subtract your age from 220 and find the range for your pulse beat between 70 and 85 percent of that number. For example, if you are 40, subtract 40 from 220 to obtain 180. Seventy percent of 180 is 126, while 85 percent is 153. During the 20-minute stimulus period, the pulse level for a person of 40 should be between 126 and 153.

Women have a slightly higher rate, so they should subtract their age from 226. If you are, for instance, 46, subtract 46 from 226. This gives you 180 as the maximum heart rate. Your exercise target rate is between 70 percent and 85 percent of 180, which gives you an upper limit of 153 on your target exercise rate.

To take your pulse, use your first two fingers (not your thumb). Press lightly on your radial artery (close to your thumb on the inside of your wrist) or on your carotid artery (straight down from the corner of your left eye, just under your chin). Health educator Dr. L. Zohman recommends counting the number of beats for 10 seconds. Multiply by six to determine the beats per minute

KNOW YOUR TARGET HEART RANGE

Your target heart range gives you a training zone of safe, effective exercise pulse rates based on your age and level of fitness. The American College of Sports Medicine recommends that you calculate both 70 percent and 85 percent of your maximum heart rate to find the low and high ends of your range. Your pulse rate during exercise will vary, but it should fall within this range.

Training Range	Sample 40-Year-Old
Start here (women start at 226)	220
Subtract age	− 40
Predicted maximum safe heart rate	180
Multiply by 0.7 for 70% (the low end of your range)	180
	× 0.7
	126
Multiply by 0.85 for 85% (the high end of your range)	180
	× 0.85
	153
After exercising, multiply your 10-second heart rate by 6 to be sure your rate per minute falls within your safe training range	25
	× 6
	150

to make sure you're within your training range.

During workouts take your pulse when you start breathing hard. If you're below your zone, work a bit harder. If you're above it, slow down. Take your pulse every 5 to 10 minutes during exercise and promptly after the aerobic workout.

This formula is a general guide. Scientific studies show that taking your pulse to determine your heart rate (as described above) isn't totally reliable. You must pay attention to your body for signs of overexertion such as pounding in the chest, dizziness, faintness, or profuse sweating.

THE WARM-UP AND COOL-DOWN

It is always a temptation to just start and stop any aerobic exercise. But regardless of how fit you are, both warm-ups and cool-downs are vital for easing the body into and out of exercise. They reduce the muscle stiffness, protect you from injuries, and make exercise itself more enjoyable.

A good warm-up results in loose, flexible muscles that are less likely to be strained or pulled than tight ones. As a result, many people begin a workout by stretching. Unfortunately you do not get much benefit stretching a cold muscle. The best way to warm up is to exercise at a light pace for a few minutes, or until you begin to perspire. Warming up like this increases the blood flow to the muscles and tendons and raises their temperature, which increases their flexibility. A warm-up also prepares your heart to meet the muscles' increased demand for blood. In one study, 70 percent of the healthy males who took stress tests experienced abnormal heartbeats during exercise if they did not warm up beforehand. Warming up eliminated the irregularities.

After you complete the training phase of your workout, cool down by slowing down. Physiologists have observed that stopping exercise abruptly can cause a sudden drop in blood pressure. You can lessen this stress by performing your exercise at a slower pace for 5 to 15 minutes until your breathing returns to normal. Ending a workout this way keeps blood flowing through working muscles, stabilizes blood pressure, and lets your heart rate descend slowly.

You can enhance any exercise period with a few stretching exercises at the end of the workout. Those described here are static stretches designed to loosen muscles gradually without straining them. Move into position slowly, hold that position for 10 to 30 seconds, relax, then repeat the stretch several times.

1. Lower leg stretch: To loosen the calf muscles and connective tissues in the feet, lean against a wall, step forward with one foot, bend the front knee, and move your hips forward. Keep your rear foot flat and your knee straight. Repeat with the other leg.

2. Quadriceps: To stretch the large muscle in the front of your thigh, brace yourself against a wall and grasp one foot. Gently pull toward your buttocks, keeping your back straight. Repeat with the other leg.

3. Groin: Sit on the ground with the soles of your feet together. Hold your toes, and gently lean forward from the waist. You should feel the stretch not only in your groin, but also in your inner thighs and lower back.

4. Hamstrings and lower back: Lie on your back. Draw one knee toward your chest while keeping the other knee flat on the ground. Grasp your knee, and gently pull it a bit farther. Repeat with the other leg.

5. Upper body: With arms extended behind you, interlace your fingers, and push up and back. Keep your chest out and your head erect. The stretch should flow down from your shoulders to your upper arms and chest.

6. Neck: Drop your head back and look straight up. Slowly roll your head to the left, then to the right. Repeat this movement, keeping your shoulders and back as straight as possible.

WHICH AEROBIC EXERCISE?

All aerobic exercises help build heart fitness. Which one you choose depends on your individual needs. Let's take a look at the advantages and disadvantages of the most popular.

Jogging

Often I am asked, "Lee, what is your favorite exercise?" Years ago I would have suggested that you join the army of joggers as I did, and for good reason. As Dr. Kenneth Cooper claims, jogging gives you the most benefit in the shortest time. But now I realize that jogging, while still extremely popular, isn't for everyone.

Today many of our popular government leaders and Hollywood celebrities are dedicated joggers. On a typical day in the Los Angeles area, you can see Charlton Heston, Robert Redford, Bess Myerson, Paul Newman, Al Pacino, and other stars huffing and puffing along their jogging trails. Former Senator William Proxmire jogs regularly, never missing a day in spite of heat, rain, or snow. His motivation, in addition to staying in good health, is the fact that his jogging burns 1,000 calories a day, helping him to keep the weight on his six-foot frame under 160 pounds. Alan Cranston, California's senior senator, who is over 60, not only jogs but participates in competitive meets. Cranston says he has always been a track nut. He ran in grade school, became a track star in high school, and had an outstanding running record in college. George Bush is a jogger, which should keep his Secret Service agents in good shape. Although jogging and running are not quite as popular as they used to be, the daily jogs of these and other well-known personalities still make it one of the most popular aerobic activities.

How well I remember starting my own jogging program over 30 years ago. My children watched in embarrassment as their old man jogged around the neighborhood in the days when it was rare to see someone running alone. Several times I was stopped by police who wanted to know why anyone in his right mind would be running through the streets unless he was being chased. It certainly is good today to hear my family brag to their friends about what good shape their father is in. I'm happy to know that at my age I can run over 25 miles without stopping to rest, while as a teenager I could barely finish a mile-long race.

A major study conducted by physiologist Dr. Harley Hartung at the Baylor College of Medicine compared the cardiovascular fitness of 22 serious joggers who averaged 18 miles a week, 22 marathoners who logged over 40 miles a week, and 22 "sedentaries" whose regular exercise was limited to such activities as walking the dog. All of those studied were middle-aged, and none was obese.

The results showed that both groups of runners were in better overall health than the sedentaries. However, while the marathoners were in better overall condition than the joggers, they had no significant advantage over the joggers in blood pressure, blood fat levels, or body weight, crucial factors for heart disease. Dr. Hartung concluded that while there may be "a minimal threshold of physical activity necessary for cardiovascular benefit," beyond that threshold the marathoners are not increasing their protection against heart attack.

Advantages: One of the advantages of jogging is that it does not require special equipment or skills; a local school ground, riverbank, or open field can provide the necessary space. Jogging, as already mentioned, gives you the most benefits in the least amount of time. It is especially valuable because it exercises the legs. When the legs move vigorously, more blood is pumped through the veins to the heart. In fact, the legs can be thought of as auxiliary pumps.

Disadvantages: Research at the Centers for Disease Control, Atlanta, found that 13 percent of male runners and 17 percent of female runners seek medical help for running-related injuries each year. After over 30 years of running, including many fun runs and an occasional marathon, the pounding on my joints has taken its toll, especially since I was one of those runners who believed "no pain, no gain."

The surface you run on, of course, is important. It goes without saying that landing on grass or soft dirt rather than concrete causes less impact on the body. Fortunately I live close to a river whose banks provide a variety of cushioned trails. I first became aware of the importance of a soft surface when I jogged indoors on a wooden floor during the rainy season. My legs developed so many aches and pains that I decided to run outside, and my soreness gradually went away. Now when I jog indoors, I run on a trampoline. By using this device I can do my aerobic exercises and give my weight-bearing joints a much-needed rest. The main reason I don't participate in more marathons is that they are held along highways and other hard surfaces, and the constant pounding of my legs leaves me in pain for several days after the race.

Fitness experts say to select jogging if you are in good physical condition, are already active, have access to a soft surface on which to jog, and enjoy running.

Swimming

A report by the President's Council on Physical Fitness and Sports recently compared the advantages of swimming to those of other sports ranging from bowling to bicycling. It rated swimming as best for building the body's stamina. Swimming equals jogging's ability to improve muscular endurance and is second only to calisthenics for increasing suppleness and flexibility. It is also superior to jogging and bicycling for developing overall body strength. Studies show no difference in the cardiorespiratory efficiency of swimmers and joggers. Dr. Jack Joseph found that either activity could condition the cardiorespiratory systems of middle-aged men and women. And a recent study at the University of Texas Health Science Center in Dallas showed that swimming can significantly improve cardiovascular function.

Advantages: Studies now show that more people swim on a regular basis than perform any other aerobic activity. Swimming exercises the entire body, toning the arms, shoulders, waistline, hips, and legs all at once. It is an excellent aerobic sport that builds endurance and strength without hurting bone and muscle. Injuries are uncommon. You don't need expensive equipment such as sports shoes.

Disadvantages: You must have access to a pool, although with the YMCA, high school, and college pools open to the public in many areas, this generally isn't a serious problem. Probably the major disadvantage is that swimming on a casual basis will not ensure a healthy heart. In some cases it is possible for a swimmer to go 20 laps a day and still not obtain much stress. Some swimmers may even reach the point where they have to swim two or three hours a day to build up stress. For this reason, swimmers should take the pulse test as they go along to make sure they are reaching the training level.

To derive maximum benefit from your swimming workouts, you can use a YMCA program called interval training. A good way to begin interval training is to swim one length of the pool at three-quarters top speed, then get out and walk back. For someone in poor or customary shape, try a routing of 10 lengths for several weeks. Walk back after each length. As you increase your endurance, increase the number of lengths gradually to 40. Change the routing by swimming one length at three-quarters speed; then, instead of walking, loaf back in the pool. You can experiment with a variety of distances and times, remembering that it is essential to alternate a period of stress with a period of recovery.

Swimming is a fine aerobic exercise no matter what your age. It is especially suited to anyone with a disability. Not long ago, I hurt my knee skiing and couldn't jog, walk, or climb stairs. Then I discovered that if I lowered myself into a pool without my feet touching the bottom, I could "jog" in place. The movement of my arms and one leg let me get a vigorous workout. The orthopedist who treated my knee injury recommends this exercise to all his patients—including many ex-joggers, ex-racquet-ballers, and ex-tennis players. Currently at Charlottes-ville, Virginia, there is a specially built 8 × 10-foot runner's pool that is available for injured people who can't exercise any other way. This is so popular that it is booked eight hours a day.

Swimming may be the best exercise for sedentary adults, who are more prone to injuries from weight-bearing exercise such as running or jogging. It may also be a good exercise for persons who have asthma or neuromuscular disorders.

Swimming is also recommended for anyone over 40 who wants to maintain aerobic fitness. Dr. Paul Hutinger, a research specialist in the physiology of exercise at Western Illinois University, calls swimming the "fountain of youth" because, unlike many forms of exercise, it easily becomes a lifetime activity.

Dr. Herbert DeVries of the University of Southern California's Andrus Gerontology Center found dramatic confirmation of the antiaging effects of swimming. Swimmers aged 50 to 87 given hour-long workouts three times a week showed profound changes after six weeks. Many of those in their seventies regained the strength and vitality they had in their fifties.

Bicycling

Dr. Clifford Graves, a California physician and founder of one of the nation's first cycling clubs, recommends cycling as a sport you can have fun with while strengthening your heart. Many experts, however, feel that a stationary bicycle probably doesn't provide enough stress for the heart unless the tension and speed can be changed. In addition, most people don't keep at it consistently enough to achieve cardiovascular fitness.

Advantages: Cycling improves the wind and slims the body. Participants also find that cycling presents fewer problems than jogging or tennis. Explains Dr. Jack Wilmore, former physiologist, University of California, Davis, "It is a much more fluid movement. And since you don't have the continual pounding, there are fewer aches and pains."

Disadvantages: To derive the maximum cardiovascular benefit from bicycling, you must more than double the time required to achieve the same effect from jogging or swimming.

For anyone, however, who wants to avoid the pitfalls of jogging yet improve the wind and slim the body, bicycling is a recommended sport. It is also recommended for anyone who wants to combine transportation with a fitness workout. Currently thousands all across the United States use bicycles for this purpose.

I employ the bicycle for short-distance transportation. Whenever I go to the store or the post office, I get on my 3-speed, and off I go. I prefer a 3-speed because it gives me more of a cardiovascular workout than the easier-to-pedal 10-speed. I was invited some time ago by a physician client to join his cycle group for a 20-mile ride. He provided me with a 10-speed bike. Since we rode on a level road, I did not feel as if I had an honest workout.

There are now hundreds of bicycle clubs across the country that offer open membership. And most communities now either have a good network of bicycle trails or are building them for the growing army of bicyclists in their area.

Aerobic Dancing

Aerobic dancing is taking the country by storm and appeals to those who find jogging a bore yet want to stay in shape. According to the National Sporting Goods Association, 24.2 million participated in aerobic dance in 1988. It combines exercise with vigorous dance routines set to music and offers a challenging workout. The program, including "jazz exercise," has picked up enthusiastic followers ranging from children to grandparents. The program usually consists of a 45-minute dance series set to music and features cardiovascular exercise as well as muscle stretching, tuning, and coordination.

Advantages: Aerobic exercise is fun and helps strengthen muscles in the upper body as well as in the legs.

Disadvantages: Many people are uncoordinated and have trouble learning the basic steps and routines. A major disadvantage is that often the exercise is performed on hardwood floors, and many participants do not have proper shoes to absorb the impact, which leads not only to discomfort and pain but to back and knee injury.

Aerobic dance is probably the best exercise for anyone who needs a group activity to become motivated. It is also useful if you find other forms of aerobic exercise boring.

Walking

Walking is now coming into its own. A recent Gallup Poll indicates that two out of three active American adults now obtain their exercise by walking. In all, 68 percent of exercising women and 56 percent of exercising men now include walking in their workouts. Surprisingly, 25 percent of these exercisers added walking to their routine within the last year.

"Walking has always been enormously underrated as a form of exercise," says Dr. Jeffrey Tanji, director of the Sports Medicine Clinic at Sacramento's University Medical Center. "In fact, walking is a tremendous way to get the benefits of aerobic conditioning. It may not seem as glamorous as running, but it's effective, less likely to cause injury, and an individual is more likely to stick with it."

About 75 percent of the people polled who began a walking program were still at it six months later. Other exercise programs, such as jogging and aerobic dancing, have a dropout rate of 75 percent. According to a survey by the National Sporting Goods Association, there are now 54 million exercise walkers, as compared to 23 million joggers and 17 million hikers.

Walking is wonderful because it is an exercise that doesn't feel like exercise. Most people know it is good for them and that it burns calories. But many walkers do not realize that it strengthens the heart and can add years to one's life in terms of heart health. The *Journal of American Medicine* reports that walking has been shown to reduce anxiety and tension and aid in weight loss. Regular walking may also help improve one's cholesterol profile, help control hypertension, and discourage osteoporosis. Physicians also generally agree that walking is the safest, most efficient exercise for the aged.

Advantages: Walking helps the circulation of the blood throughout the body. As the muscles in the legs move, they squeeze the nearby veins, forcing the blood back to the heart, giving the feeling of well-being.

Disadvantages: Sometimes the cumulative stresses of walking can result in pain along the shin (shinsplints); Achilles tendinitis, which causes pain or tightness along the back of the ankle; pain in the instep; or heel spurs. Usually these injuries begin as minor soreness in the soft tissues such as muscles or tendons and give you plenty of warning. Never walk with pain—consult your doctor. Early treatment is neither expensive nor extensive. Appropriate walking shoes will minimize your chances of injury.

To get a training effect with walking without getting hurt or frustrated, follow the "rule of 10 percent." Start out with a comfortable distance, say 20 blocks. If you feel achy or tired, cut back 10 percent and walk 18 blocks for each of the next three days. Then increase 10 percent; walk 20 blocks for three days. If you can do it comfortably, increase another 10 percent for three days. Keep increasing by 10 percent every three days. At some point you won't have time to keep adding distance. When this happens, get your increases by walking 10 percent faster. You can fine-tune this. Increase distance by 5 percent and your speed by 5 percent. If you feel uncomfortable, cut back by 10 percent and work back up again in 10 percent increments.

Remember, to get an aerobic training benefit from walking you should reach your target rate of 70 percent of your maximum heart rate. Even if you don't, though, you can still improve your aerobic fitness, as it has been found that even low-intensity exercise reduces the risks of heart disease and cancer.

Here are some tips for taking that first step:

1. Motivation is crucial. Do whatever it takes to get yourself out the door. Sometimes it helps to schedule a walk with family or friends.

2. Make a personal commitment to walking. Develop a winning attitude by recognizing how much better you'll feel about yourself. It is vital to make walking a regular part of your life. The goal is three times a week for about 30 minutes.

3. Pick a time to walk that's right for you. Most walkers prefer the early morning hours before work. But if your schedule doesn't accommodate this, choose another time and stick with it.

4. Take advantage of walking as a means of transportation, the way to get to work or the store. This way you can get 30 minutes a day, five days a week, without any pain at all.

5. If you walk at night, carry a flashlight, wear reflective gear, and walk with others.

6. Walk within your range. Keep increasing the amount of time you walk and your energy level while walking, so you're always spending 20 minutes in your target range.

7. Make walking fun. Many people stop because they become bored with walking. You need to walk in an area such as a park, so that you look forward to your outing as a time to relax and look around.

Stair Climbing

How good is stair climbing as an aerobic exercise? In a study by Stanford University professor of epidemiology Dr. Ralph S. Paffenbarger, 16,936 Harvard alumni who attended college between 1915 and 1950 were asked what condition their heart was in, how many flights of steps they climbed, how many blocks they walked, and what type of sports they participated in. The study found that men who climbed fewer than five flights of stairs per day had a 25 percent greater chance of a heart attack than those who climbed more than five a day.

A more recent study, reported on by Michael Yessis, Ph.D., a professor of physical education at California State University, Fullerton, shows that burning 2,000 calories a week in activity, including stair climbing, may add one or two years to your life.

Dr. Yessis has developed the following aerobic stair-climbing exercise to help prevent cardiac disease. If you have been sedentary for six months or more, start with this exercise for about 20 minutes, one or two times a week. The ultimate goal will be to climb for a minimum of 20 minutes, three to five times a week, at a heart rate that keeps you within your training level.

For the first 2 weeks, walk slowly up and down 2 flights of stairs (a flight is 8 stairs). The following week, increase to 4 to 5 flights. If you don't feel stiff or sore, increase to 5 to 6 flights the next week. If you have difficulty, go back to 4 to 5 flights for an additional week. Add a flight a week until you are walking up and down 8 flights.

You don't need to change this routine until you can walk up and down for 20 to 30 minutes a day three times a week, and then you can work up to a new goal of 6 flights up and down progressively. That is, walk up 2 flights then down 2 flights, repeating 10 times. Step this up by walking up 3 flights and down 3 flights 10 times, then up 4 and down 4 flights 10 times, and finally 6 up and 6 down 10 times.

Advantages: This exercise is especially good for busy people who want to combine exercise with their daily lifestyle. It's also good because climbing stairs does not depend on good weather outside, and can easily be adapted to traveling. For example, I use the stairs of hotel fire exits for my workouts when I am on trips. A consistent stair-climbing program develops the strength and firmness of leg and buttock muscles. As you walk up and down stairs, the quadriceps (muscles on the front thighs) are continuously contracted.

Disadvantages: People who climb stairs are subject to delayed-onset muscle soreness . . . muscle pain that strikes when you've overdone it.

Rope Skipping

Skipping rope can provide a good workout in a brief amount of time. Dr. Leonore Zohman found equal cardiovascular benefit in 10 minutes of vigorous rope jumping and 30 minutes of jogging. If you decide to try jumping rope, remember it is vital to progress slowly, build up, and cool down gradually after a workout.

Cross-Country Skiing

In snowbelt states, many exercise enthusiasts have discovered that cross-country skiing provides many of the same benefits as running. Cross-country skiers have the highest maximal oxygen uptake values ever recorded and burn off 700 calories per hour.

Having gone cross-country skiing many times, I find that it requires a vigorous movement of both arms and legs and has the potential for developing physical fitness. When we spend our winter holiday in the snow country, I look forward to getting my workout and feel guiltless when I leave my running shoes at home. I think my legs also appreciate the change, since cross-country skiing is a "soft" sport in which there is no pounding, just easy kicking and gliding. Cross-country skiing keeps the heart pumping so that the runner will be in shape when he or she resumes regular exercise routines.

Isometrics and Weight Lifting

Neither isometrics nor weight lifting increases cardiovascular fitness. Isometric exercises push one side of the body against the other without producing motion. They tend to raise the blood pressure, increasing the heart's work load. Weight lifting, too, doesn't use the large muscle groups as jogging does. Several studies of the effects of weight lifting showed no significant increase in either cardiovascular or respiratory fitness. Dr. Jere Mitchell and his colleagues at the University of Texas Health Science Center at Dallas have shown that, unlike running, weight lifting can cause abnormal thickening of the heart's walls. The thick hearts found in weight lifters were similar to—though not as thick as—those often found in people with chronic high blood pressure.

If you are considering using steroids for any of your exercise activities, don't. This seems like strange advice to give anyone interested in heart health, but research shows that steroid use is still rampant among athletes. The *Journal of the American Medical Association* (*JAMA*) reported that they are in use by young people too: 6.6 percent of American 12th-grade students surveyed had used steroids. According to Professor Jay Kaplan at Wake Forest University's Gray School of Medicine, steroids increase the overall cholesterol level and suppress HDL ("good" cholesterol), create an elevated heart rate, and promote the buildup of plaque in coronary arteries.

Exercise Equipment

A recent survey by the American Sporting Goods Dealers Association shows that nearly 30 million Americans work out on exercise equipment. In 1988 Americans spent a whopping $332.4 million on stationary bikes, $129 million on treadmills, $92.5 million on rowers—the "big three" in home equipment purchases, according to a study by the Sporting Goods Manufacturers Association. Put a committed person on one of these machines or other well-made fitness equipment designed for aerobic work and healthy results will occur. A 20–30-minute workout at least three days a week will burn up fat, tone muscles, and provide a good all-around feeling. For those of you who have developed problems from years of running or other activities and want to get a good cardiovascular workout, home exercise, according to Bob Goldman, may be the answer. The choices are many.

Stationary bikes are a wise choice for those who have been inactive, are overweight, and are on a tight schedule. Bikes with computerized or electronic settings for resistance allow you to set a consistent controlled load from workout to workout. On the older manual-style bikes, it is difficult to set a consistent tension. Flywheel bikes are a recent adaptation without gears and chains. These bikes will not rock back and forth when pedaled. For aerobic exercise, the upright stationary cycle is better than the recumbent cycle. Price range: $300 to $1500.

Cross-country ski machines give a challenging aerobic workout. They take about 20 minutes to get used to but will provide you with an effective upper- and lower-body workout. These machines are safe for the injury-prone exerciser. The smooth, gliding motion puts little stress on your ankles, knees, other joints, and back. Price range: $300 to $700.

Rowing machines provide aerobic exercise and help condition both the upper and lower body. These machines require you to learn correct form and technique before getting into heavy training. You can injure your lower back by rowing too quickly with too much resistance. The preferred choice is either hydraulic or electronic. Electronic models allow you to control your resistance and keep it consistent. Price range: $300 to $600.

Treadmills are ideal for those who do not want to depend on good weather. They also eliminate the problem of being threatened by dogs or muggers. Treadmills create less impact than concrete or asphalt. You do not, however, want to use a treadmill if you have a history of impact injuries such as shinsplints, knee problems, or ankle weakness. Stay away from old-fashioned manual machines, and purchase an electronic treadmill in which the tread is moved by a motor. For an aerobic workout, you do not need an electronic display that records calories burned, speed, and workout comparisons. Models should have an emergency switch, railing, and side-runners—space on either side of the tread wide enough to place your feet when getting off. Price range: $1,500 to $5,000.

Stair-climbing simulators work the buttocks more than other machines. The up-and-down motion keeps your heart rate up while firming your posterior. Used improperly, however, these simulators aggravate the lower back. As you step, you waddle from side to side, which causes the spine to move in an unnatural way. Also, according to James M. Fox, M.D., a member of the Southern California Orthopedic Institute in Van Nuys, California, stair-climbing, equivalent to carrying four to six times the body weight, may aggravate knee conditions. If you have the strength and stamina to stand upright and are free from back and knee problems, a stair-climbing simulator can be good for you. Top models contain a computer chip offering a variety of challenging workouts. Price range: $300 to $800.

To stick with the program you choose, it is most important to select one you truly enjoy. Otherwise, your equipment will just end up gathering dust in the basement.

WHICH EXERCISE FOR YOU?

Activity	Calories per Hour	Aerobic Yes	No	For What Lifestyle?
Aerobic dance	268			Any age. Can be strenuous, depending on level.
Carpet sweeping	94		X	OK if short on time. The more you keep moving, the better. OK for all ages.
Cycling, 6 mph	740		X	All ages. Good for active people. If inexperienced, start slowly.
Cycling, 12 mph	410		X	To middle age. Experienced cyclers only. Must be in good physical shape.
Gardening				Useful exercise for
(digging)	254		X	anyone. Especially
(mowing)	200		X	good for formerly
(raking)	107		X	inactive seniors.

Activity	Calories per Hour	Aerobic Yes	Aerobic No	For What Lifestyle?
Golf (walking)	105		X	Better than no exercise. Excellent for seniors and businesspeople who would not otherwise be active.
Hiking	247	X		Good aerobic exercise for healthy people of all ages. This option often not available locally, often not convenient to do three times a week.
Horseback riding (gallop)	180		X	Active individuals. Nonaerobic, but better than no exercise.
House painting	150		X	Useful for generally inactive people who want to keep active.
Jogging, 5½ mph	660	X		Should be active and in reasonable shape.
Jogging, 7 mph	920	X		For experienced joggers.
Racquetball (advanced)	400	X	X	Can be aerobic, but lots of starts and stops. Good for business-people, but must be in good shape.

Activity	Calories per Hour	Aerobic Yes	Aerobic No	For What Lifestyle?
Running in place	650	X		Useful for businesspeople who travel.
Running, 10 mph	1280	X		Experienced runners only.
Scrubbing floors	204		X	For anyone who wants to remain active but has little time.
Skiing (cross-country)	700	X		Good for active individuals.
Swimming				A fine exercise for almost anyone, any age.
25 yds/min	275	X		
50 yds/min	500	X		
Tennis	400		X	Good exercise for young and old. Too many starts and stops to be good aerobic exercise, but helps keep busy people active.
Volleyball	101		X	Active individuals only. Good beach exercise.
Walking, 2 mph	240	X		Good beginners' aerobic exercise. Fine for seniors.
Walking, 3 mph	320	X		
Walking, 4½ mph	440	X		
Waterskiing (novice)	165		X	Fine for active individuals.
(advanced)	222		X	Active and skilled waterskiers.

Activity	Calories per Hour	Aerobic Yes	Aerobic No	For What Lifestyle?
Window cleaning	124		X	Good for a weekend exercise.

The calories spent in the activies listed vary in proportion to body weight. They are quoted for a 150-pound person. A lighter person burns fewer calories, and a heavier person, more. For example, for a 100-pound person, reduce the calories by ⅓. For a 200-pound person, increase by ⅓. If you exercise harder or faster, you will only slightly increase the calories spent. A better way is to exercise longer and/or covering more distance.

EXERCISE YOUR OPTIONS

Recent research shows that you don't have to engage in structured activities to derive the health benefits of exercise. Scientists studying exercise conclude that there are heart benefits in all kinds of activity. It's not so much what you do as long as you're active.

One landmark long-term study of nearly 17,000 Harvard alumni, aged 35 to 74, shows that those who burned an additional 2,000 activity calories per week had longer life spans than those who burned fewer than 500 extra calories per week. Over a 6- to 10-year period, 572 of these men who burned fewer than 500 calories suffered heart attacks, 257 fatal. Heart attack rates declined with increasing activities. The conclusion was that the more calories burned in total activity, the less risk of heart attack. The protective effect of activity seemed to hold regardless of risk factors including smoking, high blood pressure, obesity, parental heart attacks, or prior athletic activity.

This means that moderate levels of activity, not necessarily structured workouts, offer these tremendous benefits: reduced risk of heart disease (a major cause of death), decreased total body fat, increased muscular strength, and joint flexibility.

FUNCTIONAL/FORMAL/FUN

If you are one of the millions of Americans who have trouble sticking to an exercise program, you may want to try increasing your activity level by adding "functional" or "fun" activities to any formal exercise program.

Formal Exercises

Formal exercises include activities you schedule on a regular basis for the purpose of improving cardiovascular fitness: jogging, aerobics, swimming, bicycling, power walking, and so on. We have already covered most of these in this chapter.

Functional Exercises

Functional exercises are physical activities that help you meet your daily needs. For example, if you ride your bicycle to work, walk to the grocery store, climb the stairs to your apartment, or push a lawn mower or vacuum, you're performing functional exercises. Even gardening offers exercise and stress-reducing benefits. I remember calling the president of a major corporation at home and being informed that he was outside working on a problem. Later he told me that whenever tension became overwhelming he would go out and work in the garden. The rising food prices that have prompted so many of us to turn to gardening may also contribute to cardiovascular improvement.

Fun Exercises

Fun exercises are recreational exercises like tennis, softball, hiking, bowling, baseball, and volleyball. Some of these come close to meeting the qualifications for a cardiovascular-aerobic exercise. I look forward to playing doubles tennis, but it doesn't provide me with much of a workout because retrieving tennis balls and resolving close calls interfere with continuity. Cardiologist Dr.

Leonore Zohman says that lunchtime tennis is not enough to build a healthy heart. However, when players are pitted against a single opponent, they average 61 percent of the maximum heart rate. That puts singles tennis just above the 60 percent cutoff established for a fitness exercise by the American College of Sports Medicine. In men's doubles, however, players average only 33 percent of the maximum possible heart rate. That leaves doubles out of the fitness category.

Golf is also considered nonaerobic and was often referred to by Dr. Paul Dudley White as nothing more than spoiling a good walk. The disadvantage of golf is that you stop too often to get a cardiovascular workout. Besides, today most golfers prefer using a golf cart. However, if you look at the oldsters such as Bob Hope who participate regularly and are in good health, it becomes apparent they are deriving some benefit.

Many of today's popular sports provide little exercise, especially for the young. Little League is a good example. Often the players spend much of their time waiting for a batter to hit the ball their way. But outside of an occasional dash around the bases, they get little real exercise. Football also is an activity that must be considered nonaerobic, since football players don't get nearly as good a workout as runners.

Your ultimate goal with exercise is aerobic fitness. The tables on pages 39–42 and 45 can help you design a program that is enjoyable and convenient by choosing fun, functional, or formal exercise as your schedule dictates. Once you include activity in you daily routine, you can improve your health, your cardiovascular fitness, and ultimately the quality of your life.

INTERVAL TRAINING

Interval training is a relatively new technique used today to improve endurance and cardiac fitness. Here's how it works. If you have been swimming at the same

FORMAL, FUNCTIONAL, OR FUN EXERCISES

Despite your daily work load, it's important to your cardiovascular health to work some calorie-burning exercise into your week. Try to stay with a regular schedule of formal aerobic exercise. If you can't, work some functional and fun activities into your week and weekend. This chart offers three different approaches to each activity.

Activity	Formal	Functional	Fun
Aerobic dancing	Aerobics class, to prerecorded audio or videotapes at home	Around home while doing housework	Going out dancing
Bicycling	Bike paths, organized group exercise	To work, to supermarket, to school	Recreational trips around neighborhood, tours
Running	On a jogging path, on a treadmill	To the supermarket, to work	Many games: basketball, soccer, tag, touch football, etc.
Swimming	Formal aerobic swimming classes, home pool aerobics	Regular swimming lessons	Scuba diving, recreational swimming, water sports
Walking	Walking groups	Mowing lawn, to work, shopping	Recreational weekend walking, hikes, golf

rate for 30 minutes a day for the last several months or years, your heart rate during exercise typically hovers between 70 percent and 85 percent of your maximum rate. When you interval train, you push your heart rate for a brief period of time above 85 percent. That is your body's aerobic threshold, the point where it switches from using mostly oxygen to using mostly other sources of energy. By pushing above that threshold, you train your body to utilize those sources more efficiently, and you postpone the point when you have to use them. If you are a runner, for instance, you sprint for, say, 30 seconds to a minute, then you return to your regular pace for several minutes to allow your body to recover. When it does, you sprint again. You repeat this cycle several times throughout your workout.

Recent research suggests that working out at an aerobic heart rate and alternating between periods of strenuous activity and less intense exercise can improve overall fitness. Dr. Arlette Perry, an exercise physiologist at the University of Miami Human Performance Laboratory, compared the fitness level of 66 college-aged women, divided into an interval group and a control group, after they participated in aerobic dance three times a week. Both groups spent 35 minutes training in the range of 75 percent to 85 percent of their target heart rate. The interval group interspersed rest periods of brisk walking with three- to five-minute intervals of aerobics, stretching the workout over a longer period of time. The control group did aerobics for 35 minutes without a break. At the end of 12 weeks, the interval group showed an 18 percent improvement in cardiovascular endurance. The steady-exercise group improved by only 8 percent.

A stationary-bike study at the University of Massachusetts yielded similar results. Two groups of cyclists covered the same mileage in a 12-minute exercise session three days a week, but the interval group rode through higher peaks and lower valleys of effort than the steady-state group. The maximum oxygen uptake (a measure of cardiovascular fitness) of the interval group improved 11 percent over 12 weeks, but the steady-state group's remained the same.

The most important variable in an interval training program is intensity. The more intense the intervals, the better, and the faster the results. But don't go over 90 percent of your maximum heart rate. Generally, tailor the interval length to the effort your sport demands—short sprints for tennis, running, and swimming; long intervals for basketball, soccer, walking, and bicycling. For general conditioning, do a mix of short, medium, and long intervals. That way you work all the body's energy systems.

Use your heart rate as a marker. If it drops to 70 percent before the end of your recovery period, start the next interval. If it hasn't dropped to 70 percent by the end of the allotted recovery time, don't begin another interval until it does. Most fitness experts recommend no more than three interval sessions a week. Good warm-up and cool-down sessions are especially important in interval workouts.

Rest as well as exercise is important. The American College of Sports Medicine recommends that you take off at least two days a week if you exercise vigorously. The body needs this quiet time to rejuvenate. If you tire easily, lose interest in working out, catch colds easily, or become injury prone, your body is telling you to slow down. Appetite loss, irritability, stress, and depression are other signals. An increased heart rate of 10 or more beats per minute over several days is another sign of overtraining.

WATCH YOUR INJURY RISK

Unfortunately there is a risk of injury in aerobic exercise, ranging from a twisted ankle to painful knee injuries and more, according to Jean Williams, Ph.D., sports psychologist and associate professor at the University of Arizona. Stressful events in your life seem to contribute to injury. By refraining from strenuous exercise during peak stress times, you can keep any risk to a minimum. During such times, you should still exercise, but be cautious.

High life stress: The following life stresses may cause you physical harm: a death in the family, moving, separation, divorce, financial disaster, and similar stressful events.

High daily stress: Watch your daily hassle quota. Your car needs a new transmission, your roommate let the dog out, you lost that big contract. None of these is long-term, but they all add up to increase your level of exercise injuries.

Lack of group support: Williams calls this low social support. You're new in town, or you've changed jobs and left friends behind. Even something as trivial as this can increase your stress level and make you more accident prone when you exercise.

Lifestyle stress: You've been eating badly and not getting enough sleep. In one study, athletes who ate three meals a day actually had fewer injuries than athletes who skipped meals. Breakfast has been proven to be particularly important.

Why does stress cause injury? When stress is present in your life, it's harder to concentrate, so you're more likely to take a wrong step or run into something or someone. Studies show that stress actually narrows your peripheral vision, so you're not fully aware of things around you.

Because you are under stress doesn't mean you must give up exercise or run the risk of injury. In fact, exercise is a great stress reducer. Just make sure you focus on your workout. Don't let your mind wander during these times, and make sure you're not doing something dangerous such as running in traffic without being aware of what's going on around you.

Physical fitness experts now believe that aerobic exercise is one of the three most important factors in any program for the prevention of cardiac disease (the others being diet and smoking). Scientists still don't understand all the mechanisms involved, but almost every day research adds another piece of information that shows that exercise increases heart health and helps you live a longer, higher-quality life.

Having been an aerobic exerciser for many years now, I believe that I am far more "heart fit" today than when I started years ago. My feelings are the same as those of Dr. Per-Olaf Astrand, world-renowned exercise physiologist and Stockholm physician, who declared, "It will take 100 years to determine the exact relationship between physical activity and premature death from coronary heart disease. But personally I can't afford to wait that long to find out, so I elect to exercise now."

3
Nutrition for
Cardiovascular Health

Over the last decade this country has undergone what might be called a nutrition consciousness revolution. About 50 percent of all Americans now say they read labels carefully before making food purchases. Many report they have eliminated or cut down on foods containing fat. Twenty-three percent say they eat less red meat; 19 percent state they drink less beer, wine, or hard liquor; and 12 percent report they consume less sugar. Twenty-one percent eat more vegetables, and 15 percent eat more fruit. The percentage who consume fish, poultry, and diet drinks is also on the rise.

Despite this rise in consciousness, many surveys still indicate that the diet of the majority of individuals continues to place them at risk for cardiac disease. Why? Because actual eating habits appear to be quite different than those reported in surveys. Many, for instance, buy and consume more vegetables while still eating a tremendous number of foods containing saturated fats. High-fat foods include salad dressings, gravies, and processed microwave foods. The rising number of two-income families has created an increase in consumption of prepared foods from delis and supermarkets. Many now eat four or five meals in restaurants each week, making it difficult to stay on a low-cholesterol diet. And children and teenagers consume increasing amounts of ice cream, candy, chocolate, cookies or doughnuts, pizza, snacks such as potato chips, and high-cholesterol fast foods.

The 1988 Surgeon General's Report on Nutrition and Health, which draws on 2,000 studies, states, "diet helped account for more than two-thirds of the 2.1 million deaths in the U.S. last year. Poor nutritional habits are strongly implicated in five of the nation's top ten killers: coronary heart disease, stroke, atherosclerosis, diabetes, and some cancers."

CHOLESTEROL

Current research to establish the role of cholesterol in heart disease began with the famous 40-year Framingham study of more than 5,000 Massachusetts residents. Clinical examinations were made every two years to measure cholesterol level, blood pressure, and other factors. Each participant underwent an electrocardiogram and a thorough cardiovascular evaluation. The study also matched clinical findings with incidence and development of heart disease.

After 10 years the study concluded that there was convincing evidence that blood cholesterol levels are related to the presence and development of coronary heart disease. Along with these conclusions, Drs. Thomas R. Dawber and Abraham Kagan also began to relate blood cholesterol levels to numbers of heart attacks. Over a 10-year period 200 participants with cholesterol levels over 260 developed heart disease. There were 140 cardiac disease cases with cholesterol levels between 240 and 260, 80 between 220 and 249, 60 between 200 and 220, and only 45 below the 200 level. Numerous other international studies support the correlation of high serum cholesterol levels and the epidemic of coronary artery disease.

What Is Cholesterol?

Cholesterol is an odorless, tasteless, waxy, white substance present in everyone's bloodstream. In small amounts it is vital to the healthy functioning of your body. It's an essential building block in cell walls and a basic ingredient in the manufacturing of hormones. Your liver makes all the cholesterol you need, so you can't develop a deficiency. Whatever cholesterol you ingest is added to your overall cholesterol level. It generally becomes a problem when your diet leaves a cholesterol surplus in your bloodstream.

But because cholesterol is an integral part of every animal cell, you ingest it every time you eat foods of animal origin. Although cholesterol is not a fat, it is fatlike in that it does not dissolve in water. Cholesterol hitches itself to bundles of lipoproteins that transport it throughout the bloodstream. As excess cholesterol circulates, it may eventually be deposited on the walls of the arteries, where it forms plaque.

In a few decades, enough cholesterol can collect on the walls to slow or block the flow of blood through the arteries, in a process called atherosclerosis, a form of arteriosclerosis, or "hardening of the arteries." Often this narrows the coronary arteries, which feed blood to the heart muscle. With flow slowed or blocked, heart pain (angina) signals that the heart muscle itself lacks enough blood to provide oxygen and enough energy to keep it pumping. Result: a heart attack.

If a blocked artery leads to hemorrhage or to a lack of blood in part of the brain, a stroke—with paralysis or loss of speech or other mental functions—can result.

Fortunately it is possible to partially reverse the effect of clogged arteries. Studies have shown that people who greatly reduce their cholesterol and fat intake and become more active can significantly reduce their blood cholesterol levels.

HDL, LDL, and Triglycerides

Cholesterol and fats move through the body attached to proteins that can dissolve in the blood. Fats are known chemically as lipids, and the fat-protein combinations are called lipoproteins, which carry triglycerides to cells, where they are used for energy or stored as fat.

The body packages cholesterol in three different forms: as HDL, LDL, and VLDL (high-density, low-density, and very-low-density lipoproteins). HDL carries excess amounts of cholesterol to the liver for recycling, helping to prevent the dangerous buildup of fatty deposits in the arteries—and thus it is referred to as the "good cholesterol." LDL and VLDL, on the other hand, the "bad cholesterols," transport cholesterol and deposit it in the tissues, including the blood vessel walls, promoting atherosclerosis. VLDL carries a huge load of triglycerides and holds more total cholesterol than does LDL. According to Sandra H. Gianturca of Baylor College of Medicine, people with high triglyceride levels also show higher VLDL levels than normal.

Generally doctors believe that the higher the HDL level, the lower the risk of coronary heart disease. Evidence has now accumulated, however, to show that coronary artery disease has more to do with a person's ratio of HDL cholesterol to his or her total cholesterol level. This relationship is shown in the table on the following page.

These ratios represent approximate risk factors for coronary artery disease. "Average risk" implies a 20 to 25 percent chance of developing coronary artery disease by age 60. Populations with a high incidence of heart disease, such as the Scots, tend to have low HDL levels, while those with a low incidence of heart disease, such as Jamaican farmers and Eskimos, have high HDL levels. Runners also tend to have a high level of HDLs.

Triglycerides are the other part of the equation. Tri-

CORONARY RISK RATES

Risk	HDL Cholesterol (mg/dl)		Ratio of Total Cholesterol to HDL Cholesterol	
	Men	Women	Men	Women
Very low (½ average)	Over 65	Over 75	Under 3.4	Under 3.3
Low risk	55	65	4.0	3.8
Average risk	45	55	5.0	4.5
Moderate risk (2 times average)	25	40	9.5	7.0
High risk (3+ times average)	Under 25	Under 40	Over 23	Over 11

glycerides are molecules of ordinary fat circulating in the blood; they always travel in association with some cholesterol. Many diseases associated with high triglyceride levels, such as diabetes and chronic kidney disease, are linked with an increased risk of heart disease. Heart attack survivors always have high triglyceride levels. A growing body of evidence implicates triglycerides in the destructive process of atherosclerosis. To offer guidelines, the National Institutes of Health recently published the following recommendations to be carried out under the direction of a physician:

• If your triglyceride levels exceed 500 milligrams per 100 milliliters of blood, reduce them with some form of treatment: diet, exercise, or medication.

• If the triglyceride levels test in the range of 250 to 500 milligrams per 100 milliliters of blood and are accompanied by other risk factors for heart disease, start treatment.

• Below 250 milligrams per 100 milliliters of blood, no treatment is necessary.

Note that a high serum triglyceride level is a more important marker for coronary artery disease risk than was previously thought, according to a reassessment of a large population study. If these results are confirmed, the clinically significant level of triglyicerides could drop from the current 500 milligrams per 100 milliliters down to about 200. Also, fasting triglyceride tests might become routine in patients with serum cholesterol levels above 200 milligrams per 100 milliliters.

Know Your Level

The National Cholesterol Education Program recommends that all adults age 20 and over be screened for high blood cholesterol. It appears that many Americans are doing so, according to a recent survey from the Food and Drug Administration (FDA). The percentage of adults who have had their blood cholesterol tested has risen from 35 percent to 59 percent since 1983.

The ideal time to have yours measured is when you are already in the doctor's office for a routine visit. Many community screening programs are also available. Inexpensive finger-prick tests are widely available at shopping malls, community centers, and health fairs. Recently a Los Angeles supermarket chain offered $8 cholesterol tests. In May 1988, a cholesterol screening program brought 400,000 people into more than 400 hospitals around the country for testing.

When having your cholesterol checked, fast for 14 hours before, and then be sure to sit down for five to ten minutes before the test; standing can cause the results to be inaccurate. Also contributing to inaccuracy is for the person taking blood to squeeze the finger. "Milking" the finger causes dilation of the blood vessel and inaccurately low test results.

The tests most often performed are "total blood cholesterol" and a lipoprotein analysis (also called a lipid profile). The total blood cholesterol measurement provides a single number that includes all the measurable cholesterol in your blood. The lipoprotein analysis provides individual results for HDL and LDL and other fatty substances in the blood.

Most experts recommend that you have the total blood cholesterol test first. If the result of your test is 200 or higher, repeat it. Though the instruments used to measure cholesterol levels are generally accurate, readings may vary as much as 5 percent, and human errors sometimes occur. Your cholesterol level also varies slightly from day to day and from season to season.

Dr. Kenneth Cooper, M.D., M.P.H., founder and clinical director of the Aerobics Center in Dallas, Texas, recommends that the average adult maintain a cholesterol level of 180 to 190. He also points out that for each percentage point you lower your blood cholesterol, you lower your risk of heart disease by roughly 2 percent. In general, though, the risk categories for cholesterol are estimated by age (see the table below).

CHOLESTEROL RISK CATEGORIES BY AGE GROUP

Risk	20–29	30–39	40 plus
Average	Below 200	Below 220	Below 240
Moderate	200–220	220–240	240–260
High	Above 220	Above 240	Above 260

"Lowering Blood Cholesterol," National Institutes of Health, Consensus Development Conference Statement.

The National Cholesterol Education Program has established the following guidelines for action based on your total blood cholesterol level (your physician may make adjustments for age, sex, heredity, background, and lifestyle):

- Total cholesterol below 200: Maintain low-cholesterol diet, minimize saturated fat. Check your blood cholesterol again within five years—sooner if there is a change in diet or a dramatic weight gain.

- Total cholesterol between 200 and 239: Have the level measured again. If it still falls within this range, begin a cholesterol-lowering diet. If you have coronary heart disease or at least two other risk factors (high blood pressure, cigarette smoking, family history of heart disease, diabetes, severe obesity, and being a male), your doctor should order a lipoprotein analysis. If your LDL level is over 130, your doctor will probably begin dietary treatment, and if it falls above 160, he or she may consider drug therapy.

- 240 and higher: Your doctor should order a lipoprotein analysis and start you on a cholesterol-lowering diet treatment. If the LDL cholesterol is over 160, your doctor should consider drug therapy as well.

Even if your lab results put you in the "safe" level, you still should not eat cholesterol-rich foods, since they increase your risk of heart disease. If you receive unfavorable results, get a second opinion before taking action.

How well I remember the results from my first lipoprotein panel, which indicated I was heading for serious trouble. I was devastated because I had spent a lifetime watching my diet. In desperation I called Dr. Peter Wood at Stanford, and he agreed to retest me in his laboratory. The new results were considerably different . . . and just about where they should be for someone who doesn't smoke, exercises daily, and consumes a low-fat diet.

My situation is not unusual. In 1985, the College of American Pathologists prepared a standardized blood sample with a cholesterol of 263 milligrams per 100 milliliters and sent it to 5,000 laboratories. The reports came back with values ranging from 197 to 397, though the majority clustered in the range of 222 to 294. Even so, a value of 222 in a middle-aged person would probably not be treated, whereas a value of 263 might be and 294 should be.

Cholesterol-Lowering Drugs
There are many cholesterol-lowering drugs, including Gemfibrozil, which reduces LDL and appears to raise HDL. Niacin, a common B vitamin, produces similar results, although it can cause side effects such as flushing and stomach disorders. Questran or Colestid are also used to lower LDL. These are resins that trap bile in the digestive tract and carry it out of the body. See the table on pages 60–61 for more information about drugs. Normally, your intestines reabsorb unused bile and reprocess the cholesterol it contains. When the resins remove the bile, they remove its cholesterol too. Because it needs cholesterol to make more bile, the liver will remove new cholesterol (especially LDL) from the blood.

The Lipoprotein Analysis
When you take a lipoprotein analysis, three substances are measured: total cholesterol, HDL cholesterol, and triglycerides. From these readings, the amount of LDL cholesterol is calculated according to a standard formula: LDL = Total Cholesterol − HDL − (Triglycerides ÷ 5).

A normal result might be a total cholesterol of 200, HDL cholesterol of 45, and triglyceride of 150. Thus the LDL level is 125, or 200 minus 45 minus 30. This formula only works if the triglyceride level is below 400. Because the triglyceride level is influenced by recent food intake, this measurement is taken before breakfast.

The level of LDL cholesterol is more closely associated with coronary risk than is total cholesterol.

LDL CHOLESTEROL

Desirable	Below 130
Borderline	130–160
High	Over 160

The Whole Story   Neither the total cholesterol nor the LDL cholesterol level tells the whole story. As described earlier, the ratio of total cholesterol to HDL cholesterol is equally important, since a person with an apparently good overall cholesterol level may have very low HDL and high LDL levels. The higher your ratio of total cholesterol to HDLs, the more your cardiovascular system is in jeopardy.

For example, if someone has a total cholesterol of 300 milligrams and an HDL count of 75, that's a ratio of 4 to 1. That person is at some risk. But if another individual has a total cholesterol of 250 and an HDL count of 25, that's a ratio of 10 to 1. That person is at higher risk even though he or she has a lower cholesterol count.

Young women are better off than young men because they tend to have an overall lower level of serum cholesterol (the level in the bloodstream) and a significantly higher ratio of HDLs. Before puberty, boys and girls have the same HDL levels. At puberty boys' HDLs fall while girls' stay unchanged because of hormonal factors. This female advantage means that men have a 10-year head start on women when it comes to the risk of heart attack. Cardiovascular disease is the leading cause of death in men over 35 and becomes the leading killer of women only after they reach 45.

Cholesterol rises with age. But in men the rate of increase slows down. Around menopause women experience an abrupt rise in cholesterol. When they reach their forties, the increase in total cholesterol jumps to two milligrams per year. And after menopause, women's LDL levels frequently skyrocket.

CHOLESTEROL-LOWERING DRUGS

Drugs	Reduced Heart Attack Risk Proven	Long-Term Safety	Easy to Take	Decrease in LDL	Side Effects	Special Precautions
Cholestyramine (Questran) Colestipol (Colestid)	Yes	Yes	No	15–30%	Constipation, stomach upset	May interfere with absorption of other drugs. May increase triglyceride levels.
Nicotinic acid (Nicamin, Nico-400, Nicobid, Nicolar, SK-Niacin, Wampocap)	Yes	Yes	No	15–30%	Flushing, heartburn, stomach upset	Not recommended for individuals with peptic ulcer, liver disease, or heart rhythm disturbances
Lovastatin (Mevacor)	No	Limited	Yes	25–40%	Infrequent gastrointestinal disturbances, muscle inflamation	Patients should be monitored for changes in liver functions and for cataracts

Gemfibrozil (Lopic)	Yes	Moderate	Yes	5–15%	Infrequent gastrointestinal disturbances	Risk of gallstones. Strengthens oral blood-thinning drugs. Occasional blood and liver changes.
Probucol (Lorelco)	No	Limited	Yes	10–15%	Infrequent gastrointestinal disturbances	Reduces HDL (good cholesterol). Not recommended for patients with heart disturbances.

National Cholesterol Education Program, *Report of the Expert Panel on Detection, Evaluation, and Treatment of High Blood Cholesterol in Adults*, 1987.

Dr. Kenneth Cooper recommends that women keep the ratio of total cholesterol to HDL cholesterol below 4.0 and men below 4.6. He also reports that 75 percent of the patients he works with can control their cholesterol by dietary restriction, exercise, and weight loss.

OBESITY

If you weigh too much, an additional work load is placed on the heart. For every pound of fat on your body, your heart has to pump blood through an extra three-quarters of a mile of blood vessels—at about 70 times a minute. Even resting, an overweight body works harder to breathe and needs more oxygen. Overweight people, even active ones, may become short of breath. And most cardiologists agree that there is at least an association between excess weight and increased risk of coronary heart disease. Dr. William B. Kannel, who directed the Framingham study, has stated that "if everyone were at optimal weight, there would be 25% less coronary heart disease and 35% less congestive failure and brain infarction."

At least one study found a significant link between how much saturated fat an individual eats and how obese he or she is, regardless of how many calories that person consumes. Besides this, a recent study by Stanford University found no correlation between how much body fat men had and the total number of calories they consumed. Instead, the most important factor was fat in the diet. Even a little fat can boost the risk of heart disease. A study of U.S. women reports that those who were slightly overweight were nearly twice as likely as lean women to experience heart attacks and angina. Those who were at least 30 percent overweight were more than three times as likely to develop heart disease.

HIGH BLOOD SUGAR

Dr. John Yudkin strongly maintains that sugar, not animal fat or cholesterol, is the big danger factor in heart disease. Dr. Yudkin and his coworkers conducted numerous laboratory tests on animals and human volunteers consuming a high-sugar diet. The diet produced many of the concomitants of heart disease, including increased cholesterol and triglyceride levels; decreased efficiency in dealing with high blood glucose, and insulin, and other hormonal disturbances; and stickier blood platelets (which contribute to clotting).

Dr. A. M. Cohen of Jerusalem found that immigrants recently arrived in Israel from Yemen, who had consumed little sugar in their native land, had little heart disease. Among the Yemenites who had emigrated 20 to 30 years earlier and had adopted the high-sugar diet of their new country, heart disease was common, and the incidence of diabetes was 50 times higher than for the new immigrants. In an unusual study, Dr. Otto Schaeffer found that Eskimos who lived near white settlements and consumed sugar had considerably more atherosclerosis than Eskimos who lived away from settlements and consumed little or no sugar. Dr. Meyer Friedman, known for his Type A/Type B classifications, also believes that sugar (especially in ice cream) deserves special attention in the search for the causes of heart disease.

Unfortunately, in today's world, it is difficult to avoid sugar. Catsup tested by a food analysis laboratory contained 29 percent sugar. Some salad dressings contain as much as 30 percent, and a coating for chicken had 51 percent. Many other foods, including peanut butter, contain similar amounts. The most common sources are sucrose, fructose, dextrose, corn syrup, invert sugar, honey, molasses, maple syrup, and brown sugar.

There are today many scientists both in and out of government who still feel sugar is safe for almost anybody and does not trigger any major disease. While awaiting the medical jury's final decision, doesn't it make sense to say no to your sweet tooth occasionally, especially when we do know that there is no physiological requirement for sugar, and all our human nutritional needs can be met without it?

EATING FOR A HEALTHY HEART

Fats

Animal fats create excess cholesterol in the bloodstream; plant fats and oils don't, with the exception of palm and coconut oils found in dairy creamers, candy bars, and similar foods. Foods high in saturated fat include butter, eggnog, ice cream, cheese, egg yolks, liver, rib-eye steak, lunch meat, bacon, creams, sauces, gravies, whipped topping, and animal organs. All cause plaque buildup, clogging the vital lifelines to the heart.

The American Heart Association recommends that we consume no more than 30 percent of our total calories from fat, divided evenly among saturated, monounsaturated, and polyunsaturated fats. Now many experts feel that we should tip the scales toward monounsaturated fats, the kind found in olive and peanut oil, because these fats lower blood cholesterol. The residents of Italy, Greece, Spain, and Portugal, where olive oil is used liberally, have a considerably lower level of heart attacks than people in countries where little olive oil is used.

Polyunsaturated fats also help lower cholesterol levels. Sources include corn, sunflower, and safflower oil, as well as certain fish oils.

Lowering Cholesterol Through Diet

To create a healthy heart Dr. Kenneth Cooper recommends a diet that consists of 60 percent complex carbohydrates, 15 percent protein, and 5 percent fat, with fewer than 300 milligrams of cholesterol a day. Such a diet, Cooper says, can yield an initial reduction in cholesterol of 13 percent in two weeks.

Experts believe that most individuals can lower their blood cholesterol by taking the following steps:

• Decrease the saturated fat in your diet until it accounts for less than 10 percent of your total caloric intake.

• Reduce your daily dietary cholesterol intake to less than 300 milligrams a day.

• Eat between 6 and 7.5 grams of soluble fiber for every 1,000 calories of food you consume each day.

To do this, start by choosing low-fat versions of foods within the major food groups: meat, dairy products, breads and cereals, vegetables and fruits.

Meat   Meat is an important group, for it is a major source of protein, which the body needs to replace dead cells and to form new ones. Everyone needs an adequate intake of protein to maintain good health and to recover from illness and injury. However, red meat poses a threat to the heart and has been associated with cancer. Studies reveal that as immigrants to the United States adopt a westernized diet with a lot of red meat, their heart attack rate rises dramatically. The rate is higher in Hawaii than in Japan and much higher in the continental United States than in Hawaii. A study of about 3,300 Chinese residents of North America and China show that people increase their risk of colon and rectal cancer when they eat a lot of saturated fat and fail to exercise. Thus, the closer these people come to our shores and the more of our diet they adopt, the higher their risk of heart attack. It's wise to look for alternatives to red meat.

Poultry and fish provide high-quality protein that is low in fat. Research shows that eating fish actually lowers cholesterol levels. Dr. William E. Connor, head of the Clinical Nutrition and Lipid Atherosclerosis Laboratory at the University of Oregon Health Sciences Center, has found that the oil found in fish can greatly lower blood levels of cholesterol and reduce the formation of blood clots.

Dr. Connor reported that in one study, after 10 days on a diet containing salmon and salmon oil, normal subjects experienced an 11 percent decrease in cholesterol levels and a 33 percent drop in triglycerides. In persons with dangerously elevated blood fat levels, the salmon and salmon oil produced a 32 percent reduction in cholesterol and a remarkable 66 percent decrease in triglycerides. As far as fish oil supplements, however, paddle the other way. It appears that fish oil is most useful when eaten with the other natural components in the fish. Fish oil supplements, too, may be harmful, as evidenced by a study at the Minneapolis Veterans Affairs Medical Center. There is a chance of overdosing on the supplements. Eating fish, on the other hand, remains a safe and apparently life promoting habit. (I personally wish President Bush would consider these "health facts" and consume more of the fish he catches on vacation, instead of his favorite food, pork rinds, which are pig skins fried in lard and salt. A two-ounce serving contains more than 50 percent fat and 58 milligrams of cholesterol. I would also like to see the President reinstate broccoli to the White House menu, in spite of his dislike for this most healthy vegetable!)

Legumes such as dried beans and dried peas do not contain the high-quality protein of meat but are often included in the meat category because of their protein content. When eaten with rice, corn, or a little lean meat, the protein contained in legumes rivals that of meat.

When selecting red meat for your diet, choose meat

with the least amount of marbling (fat mingled among muscle tissue) and the least amount of visible fat. Always buy the leanest ground beef available, and pour off the fat after browning it. Trim visible fat from meat. Bake or broil instead of frying. Skim the fat off meat juices before adding them to stews, soups, and gravy.

Eat only small amounts of liver, tongue, kidneys, sweetmeats, heart, brains, or chitterlings. They are high in cholesterol. When the body consumes animal organs, the cholesterol they contain is absorbed directly into the bloodstream during the digestive process. Although liver is high in cholesterol, it can be used in small amounts occasionally, because it is a good source of iron.

Milk and Milk Products   Some nutritionists recommend switching from butter to margarine and liquid vegetable oils, but others question this substitution. Cheeses also should be consumed with caution. Cheddar, Muenster, and Swiss cheeses, for instance, derive 70 to 80 percent of their calories from fat. And two slices of American cheese contain almost as much fat as a Quarter Pounder. For cheese lovers, however, there are now cheeses in supermarkets that contain one-half to two-thirds of the fat and half the cholesterol of cheddar, Swiss, and similar types, as well as considerably less salt and 30 percent more calcium.

Breads and Cereals   As if we don't have enough diet decisions to make, I recently counted over 50 brands of bread in my favorite supermarket. Since bread truly is the staff of life, the decision is a vital one. If yours is a typical American family, each of you will have a slice of toast for breakfast, two slices of bread in a sandwich for lunch, and perhaps another slice of bread or a roll for dinner. Because bread is so common and so vital in our diet, we need guidance in making a wise choice.

First, reject all brands that have either preservatives or additives. Next, eliminate those from which the most nutritious parts of the wheat kernel have been removed. The kernel is made up of three parts. The first is the outer covering, or bran, a rough, many-layered shield rich in crude fiber. Next comes the starchy mass called the endosperm. Deep inside is the tiny embryo, or wheat germ, which Mother Nature has wisely provided with all the nutrients needed to spark growth into a new wheat plant. This wheat germ contains the entire B vitamin complex, plus zinc and magnesium. Wheat germ actually contains more than 26 percent protein with no saturated fat. T-bone steak, on the other hand, contains only 19 percent protein with lots of fat.

White bread is made from the endosperm, the least nutritious part of the kernel, with the bran and the wheat germ thrown away. White flour was being produced in Greece at least as early as 500 B.C., and by A.D. 50 its production was widespread. By the end of the seventeenth century everyone was eating it. Bakers now try to tempt us to eat bread made from white flour by claiming it is "enriched." While several vitamins and minerals are added, they do not make up for all the lack of nutrition in this product. Whole-wheat flour, on the other hand, contains the nutrition of all parts of the kernel.

Fruits and Vegetables   Several studies report that foods from the vegetable and fruit group can cause a fall in blood cholesterol levels, possibly because they decrease the levels of saturated fatty acids or because they contain generous amounts of pectin and fiber. Pectin, a carbohydrate, is found in the skins of many fruits as well as in vegetables and sunflower seeds. Eating two carrots a day will help to lower cholesterol levels—as with oat products, it's the soluble fiber that is believed to be responsible for the beneficial effects. Many nutritionists advocate a vegetarian diet or a diet with little meat and few animal products to manage plasma lipid levels of some patients (those capable of making the necessary changes).

Onions, garlic, and other members of the onion family have also been especially recommended by some nutritionists for their cholesterol-lowering properties. Studying groups of vegetarians, D. S. Sainai of the B. J. Medical College in Poona, India, found low levels of cholesterol in those who ate large amounts of garlic and onions, moderate levels in those who consumed moderate amounts of these vegetables, and higher cholesterol levels in those who ate neither onions nor garlic. Dr. Arun Bordia also found that garlic distinctly inhibited blood clotting.

Most fruits are rich sources of vitamin C, which can lower blood cholesterol, preventing the onset of atherosclerosis. While fruit juices are recommended, they do not measure up to whole fruit. An orange, for example, supplies three times more fiber than six ounces of orange juice. An apple without the peel contains five times more fiber than six ounces of apple juice.

Without a doubt fruit juices are preferable to soft drinks, which contain no nutrient value and an excess amount of sugar. Unfortunately, the consumption of soft drinks continues to skyrocket. According to the Coca-Cola Company, soft-drink consumption has grown at an annual rate of approximately 95 percent over the last 20 years. And today soft drinks account for approximately 30 percent of all commercial beverage consumption. To make matters worse, some companies have promoted this product as a breakfast drink.

A Cholesterol-Reducing Diet

Current research now shows that you can lower your cholesterol by carefully selecting the foods you eat. An easy way to make sure you eat the right foods is to divide each food into three subgroups by the amount of saturated fat or the amount of fiber particular foods

LOVE-YOUR-HEART FOOD LIST

Food	Portion	Calories	Grams of Saturated Fat	Grams of Soluble Fiber
Meat Group A				
Chicken (white meat, no skin)	3.5 oz.	140	0.4	—
Cod	3.5 oz.	168	0.2	—
Kidney beans	1 cup	230	—	3.0
Lobster	3.5 oz.	95	0.1	—
Salmon	3.5 oz.	66	2.0	—
Turkey (white meat)	3.5 oz.	175	0.5	—
Tuna (in water)	3.5 oz.	125	1.5	—
Meat Group B				
Beef, round steak	3.5 oz.	259	3.0	—
Ground beef, lean	3.5 oz.	217	7.0	—
Leg of Lamb, lean	3.5 oz.	266	3.0	—
Sausage, pork	3.5 oz.	494	3.0	—
Meat Group C				
Bacon	3.5 oz.	578	17.5	—
Frankfurter, beef	2.0 oz.	458	12.9	—
Milk Group A				
Cottage cheese	3.0 oz.	90	0.5	—
Milk, skim	8.0 oz.	44	0.3	—
Yogurt, plain	8.0 oz.	113	0.2	—
Milk Group B				
Cheese, whole-milk	1.0 oz.	115	5.0	—
Milk, whole (3.5% fat)	8.0 oz.	80	5.0	—
Yogurt, fruit	8.0 oz.	150	5.0	—

Milk Group C				
Ice cream	1 cup	165	14.5	—
Mayonnaise	1 tbsp.	101	1.5	—
Pie, chocolate cream	⅛ pie	265	17.0	—
Vegetable Group A				
Broccoli	½ cup	27	—	1.0
Corn, cooked	½ cup	192	—	1.5
Peas	½ cup	58	—	2.0
Potato, baked, medium	1 potato	92	—	2.0
Vegetable Group B				
Carrots, raw	½ cup	96	—	0.5
Lettuce	½ cup	13	—	0.2
Tomato, raw	1 medium	92	—	0.2
Vegetable Group C				
Avocado	1 medium	369	5.0	—
Grain Group A				
Bread, whole-wheat	1 slice	76	—	3.0
Cornmeal	1 cup	433	—	4.0
Oat bran, dry	1 cup	255	—	6.0
Oatmeal, cooked	1 cup	132	—	2.0
40% bran flakes	1 cup	106	—	1.0
Flour, all-purpose	1 cup	419	—	2.0
Tortillas, corn	1 tortilla	65	—	1.0
Grain Group B				
Spaghetti, cooked	1 cup	182	0.5	0.5
Bread, white	1 slice	76	0.3	—
Grain Group C				
Angel food cake, enriched	⅙ cake	161	0.2	—

contain. The Love-Your-Heart Guide dietary suggestions listed in the table on pages 70–71 are divided this
way. The dairy and meat items are rated for their saturated fat content. Dairy foods and meats with the least
amount of saturated fat are in the A group, those with
moderate amounts of saturated fat in the B group, and
those with the highest saturated fat content in the C
group. Fruits and vegetables and grain products are
graded by their fiber content. Those with the highest
fiber content are in the A group, those with moderate
fiber content in the B group, and those with little fiber
in the C group. Avocados and olives contain so much fat
they are placed in the C category.

The table below will help you establish an allowable
daily intake of saturated fat (10 percent or less of total
caloric intake). Select foods from the Love-Your-Heart
meat and milk food list (pages 70–71), keeping the total
saturated fat intake at or below your daily minimum.

For instance, if you are a woman who weighs 120
pounds, you need to eat 18 or fewer grams of saturated

TOTAL GRAMS OF SATURATED FAT
ALLOWABLE PER DAY

Men Desirable Weight (in pounds)	Total Grams	Women Desirable Weight (in pounds)	Total Grams
100	17	100	15
120	20	120	18
140	23	140	21
160	27	160	24
180	30	180	27
200	33	200	30

Official U.S. Government and U.S. National Academy of Science
recommends that total fat in our diets be limited to 30% of calories.

fat every day. However, if you eat 3.5 ounces of bacon for breakfast and 2 hot dogs for lunch, you have already consumed 29.5 grams of saturated fat that particular day . . . 9.5 grams over the target goal.

As already explained in the table on pages 70–71, all meat and milk items in section A are low in saturated fat, all items in section B contain moderate amounts of saturated fat, and items in section C are high in saturated fat. If you select 60 to 70 percent of your food from section A, 25 to 30 percent from section B, and only 5 to 10 percent from section C, you will easily stay within your target range for saturated fat.

That's half the picture. The other half is the fiber in your diet. Generally you need to eat between 6 and 7.5 grams of soluble fiber every day. All plant foods contain fiber, some of it soluble, some insoluble. While both kinds are good for you, in terms of lowering blood cholesterol the insoluble fiber is more effective. The table on pages 70–71 shows you the soluble fiber content for various fruits, vegetables, and grains. Section A foods contain the most fiber, section B moderate amounts, and section C small amounts (and in some cases contain fats). By selecting 65 to 70 percent of your foods from vegetable and grain group A, 25 to 30 percent from group B, and 5 to 10 percent from group C, you will obtain all the fiber you need.

Counting Dietary Cholesterol

To lower your blood cholesterol you must limit the cholesterol you consume to less than 300 milligrams a day. This does not mean counting daily cholesterol consumption. As long as you meet your daily targets for saturated fat and fiber, you almost automatically meet this requirement. That's because foods low in saturated fat and high in soluble fiber tend to be low in cholesterol. The exceptions are liver, shrimp, and eggs. All are low in saturated fat but high in cholesterol. One egg and a little liver is all the cholesterol you need for one day.

CHOLESTEROL CONTENT OF BASIC FOODS

Food	Cholesterol (in milligrams)
Fruits, grains, vegetables	0
Scallops (cooked, about 3½ oz.)	53
Oysters (cooked, about 3½ oz.)	45
Clams (cooked, about 3½ oz.)	65
Fish, lean (cooked, about 3½ oz.)	65
Chicken/turkey, light meat (without skin, cooked, about 3½ oz.)	80
Lobster (cooked, about 3½ oz.)	85
Beef, lean (cooked, about 3½ oz.)	90
Chicken/turkey, dark meat (without skin, cooked, about 3½ oz.)	95
Crab (cooked, about 3½ oz.)	100
Shrimp (cooked, about 3½ oz.)	150
Egg with yolk, one	213
Beef liver (cooked, about 3½ oz.)	440
Beef kidney (cooked, about 3½ oz.)	700

Center for Medical Consumers, *Health Facts* 12, no. 93 (1987): 2.

Eating Out

Anyone who eats out regularly knows that the food choices offered in restaurants make it difficult to stay on a heart-healthy diet. Some fast-food chicken sandwiches contain as much fat as one and a half pints of ice cream. Chicken nuggets, if cooked in fat, have as much fat as a hamburger. Salads present their own problems. If you load your plate with potato and pasta salads, bacon, and creamy dressings, your salad will have more fat than a quarter-pound cheeseburger. A three-ounce serving of carrot and raisin salad contains 198 calories and four teaspoons of fat. Tuna salad has 156 calories and two teaspoons of fat.

With care, you can still eat out and stay on a healthy diet. A good salad choice is three ounces of mixed vegetables (including onions and carrots) and lettuce. A teaspoon of low-calorie dressing has virtually no fat and is under 50 calories. In many restaurants special-order menus offer low-salt, low-fat, low-cholesterol meals that are both healthy and delicious. Since you cannot read labels as you can at home, be aware of which items are high in saturated fat.

Supermarket Shopping

Sometimes when shopping it's a little difficult to tell which foods are heart healthy and which aren't. Here are a few tips to guide your supermarket searches.

To compare foods, you should know how much fat each contains, not just how much fat is saturated. That's because all fats are a mixture of saturated and unsaturated fatty acids. For example, even soybean oil is 15 percent saturated, so a tablespoon contains 14 grams of fat of which 2 grams are saturated.

Some breakfast cereals boast that they contain only 1 gram of fat per half-cup serving. However, often the fat is coconut or palm oil, tropical oils which, although cholesterol-free, are fats to be avoided because they are high in saturated fat. And saturated fat can do more to raise your cholesterol level than dietary cholesterol itself. If a label says "cholesterol-free," be sure to check the type of oil in the food.

A clear rule of thumb is, of course, the less fat the better. And if a food contains no more than one or two grams of fat, it really doesn't matter whether the fat is saturated or unsaturated.

Watch out for foods that have special labeling rules. For instance, ground beef labeled "lean" or "extra lean" has more fat than the Department of Agriculture allows in other meat or poultry products labeled "lean" or "extra lean." According to the USDA, "lean" meat or poultry can be no more than 10 percent fat, and "extra lean" means no more than 5 percent fat. But the USDA ex-

CALORIES, FAT, AND SODIUM IN FROZEN ENTREES

Product (serving)	Calories	Fat (%)	Sodium (mg)
LEAN			
Benihana Lite Dinners (9 oz.)	250	14	1,096
Light & Elegant (9 oz.)	264	18	859
Benihana Classic Dinners (11 oz.)	319	20	1,321
Chun King Entrees (10 oz.)	290	20	1,250
Armour Dinner Classics (11 oz.)	260	23	871
Le Menu Light Style Dinners (12 oz.)	262	25	680
Mrs. Paul's Light Seafood (10 oz.)	259	26	796
Stouffer Lean Cuisine (10 oz.)	261	28	934
FATTIER			
Green Giant (10 oz.)	334	31	1,104
Budget Gourmet Slim Selects (10 oz.)	283	32	831
Old El Paso Mexican Dinners (13 oz.)	388	32	1,158
FATTY			
Swanson Hungry-Man Entrees (12 oz.)	520	40	1,398
Celentano (10 oz.)	327	40	484
Le Menu Dinners (11 oz.)	401	42	985
Swift International Entrees (6 oz.)	358	42	865
Swanson Hungry-Man Dinners (17 oz.)	705	43	1,639
Barber Foods (7 oz.)	426	47	957
Stouffer Entrees (10 oz.)	356	48	1,068
Banquet Dinners	719	50	1,243
Le Menu Entrees	355	51	783
Swanson Entrees	350	54	833

empts ground beef. The average "lean" ground beef sold in stores is 21 percent fat. The average "extra lean" is 17 percent fat. If you want truly lean ground beef, buy ground round steak. Similarly, 2-percent milk can be labeled "low-fat" even though it has more fat than the FDA allows in other "low-fat" foods.

Oils, margarines, Tofutti, and many other foods labeled "low cholesterol" are not low in fat. Also beware of claims and labels that don't tell the whole story. The meat industry often claims that beef has no more cholesterol than chicken, which is true, but it is also true that beef has more saturated fat than chicken.

Although it takes a little effort to stay on a heart-healthy diet under all conditions, it is well worth the effort.

A nutritious diet is a vital part of any program for preventing cardiac disease. Generally, however, there is no need to do any complicated counting. Learn which foods make up the A groups, which the B, and which the C. Then, whether you are eating at home or dining out, simply select those foods that help keep you within your target range. To quote a recent study in *Postgraduate Medicine*: "The prevalence of high serum cholesterol levels and the associated epidemic of coronary artery disease are largely the by-products of a maladaptive diet."

Nutrition is an important factor in preventing cardiac disease, and with proper eating habits you can begin to control this risk almost automatically.

4
Reducing High Blood Pressure

You have no pain, nor do you feel sick, yet you could very well be walking around with hypertension—the medical term for high blood pressure—the primary cause of about 60,000 deaths a year. It is also the contributing factor in a million deaths annually from stroke and other types of heart disease.

In most cases there are no symptoms. In a few instances, high blood pressure shows up in the form of persistent headaches, dizziness, fatigue, or shortness of breath. Although it is clearly a significant problem, it can be detected early, and treatment is available.

WHO'S AT RISK?

Basically, the older you are, the greater the risk. Under age 50, hypertension is more common in men than in women. After age 55 or 60, women show a higher increase than men . . . yet more men die from the complications of high blood pressure than do women. While it still is not known how common this problem is among school-aged youngsters, a study of Dallas children showed that close to 9 percent of 10,000 eighth graders have elevated blood pressure. In addition a recent British study showed that the incidence of high blood pressure is increasing among adolescents and that the readings rise with age. Having a child's blood pressure taken is the first step in preventing adult hypertension, because hypertension for some people begins in childhood.

CONTRIBUTING FACTORS

The tendency to develop high blood pressure appears to be genetic. If other members of your family suffer from high blood pressure, you probably are at high risk to develop hypertension.

In addition, blacks show a greater tendency toward high blood pressure than do whites. A recent study found that almost 50 percent of blacks over age 65 are hypertensive, while only 25 percent of whites in this age group have high blood pressure. A number of theories have been advanced to explain this, including the high salt content of soul food and the stress associated with being a minority subjected to prejudice. A University of Michigan study deemphasizes genetic factors among blacks and points instead to the levels of stress in the areas where blacks live. The blood pressures of black men and women in low-stress Detroit neighborhoods consistently tested eight to nine percentage points lower than the blood pressure of blacks from high-stress neighborhoods.

Certain personality types also show tendencies toward hypertension. Studies of air force officers describe those with the highest blood pressures as "dominant, assertive and decisive, with narrow ranges of interest, over-controlling, rigid, and obtuse in social relationships." In addition, an insurance company employee survey found that people with high blood pressure were "guarded, apprehensive, and unwilling to talk about themselves."

Since the 1930s researchers have suggested a link between suppressed anger and hypertension. More recently a number of different laboratory approaches have been used to investigate this connection. The studies concluded that individuals with high blood pressure have difficulty acknowledging angry feelings and are not likely to express anger overtly. Currently studies indicate that suppressed hostility may have as great an effect on blood pressure as other more commonly acknowledged risk factors.

Besides this, stressful occupations and environments have turned out to be a contributing cause. A 1986 study of 1,500 San Francisco city bus drivers showed that 40 percent of the drivers had high blood pressure, twice the incidence of any other group—a problem shared by transit workers worldwide.

Other studies indicate that hypertension is a disease of civilized life . . . answering part of the question as to why many seemingly calm and even-tempered people develop high blood pressure when thrust into a hostile environment.

WHY IS HIGH BLOOD PRESSURE A THREAT?

Think for a moment of the circulatory system as a vast network of hollow tubes like a garden hose, with the heart as the master pump. Like cholesterol, blood pressure in itself is not bad. In fact, it is essential because a certain amount of pressure is needed inside the miles of blood vessels to push the blood, with the nutrients and oxygen it carries, to every cell in the body.

Since blood vessels are soft and elastic, they can stretch and contract to control the flow of blood through them. However, when something causes the pressure to soar, there is a tremendous strain on their walls.

When vessels stay open, blood flows freely, and little pressure builds up on the artery walls. Problems arise if the vessels are constricted or closed. To push the blood through these obstructions in order to reach the brain, kidneys, and other parts of the body, the heart must pump harder; like any overworked muscle, it becomes enlarged and thickened, and its fibers become overstretched. Eventually it fails to function as an effective pump. The problem doesn't stop there. The stretching of the artery walls can begin to destroy the elastic fibers, or make them hard, brittle, and less elastic.

The Bottom Line

Eventually this causes a number of problems. Here is a rundown of the most serious.

High blood pressure tends to cause hardening of the arteries, as deposits of minerals and cholesterol build up inside the arteries, narrowing the passageway and preventing the blood from flowing normally. When this plaque becomes large enough to completely obstruct the coronary artery, it can create a sudden decrease in the oxygen supply to the heart. In addition, plaque can break away and lodge farther along in the artery, again restricting oxygen to the heart and causing a heart attack. This killer (called an occlusion) often strikes without warning.

Stroke   A stroke occurs when the blood supply is cut off by blockage or rupture of the blood vessels that supply oxygen to the brain. When this supply line is interrupted, brain cells denied their energy-giving blood source begin to die. As a result, the functions they control—speech, muscle movement, memory, or comprehension—may die with them. This effect is called a stroke or, in medical terms, a cerebrovascular accident (CVA).

A blockage can result from a thrombus, the medical word for a blood clot that develops at the site of the blockage, or an embolus, a clot that develops elsewhere in the body and travels until it lodges in the brain's supply lines. Fatty buildup, called plaque, in the lining of the arteries can narrow the passageway through which blood travels, making clotting more likely to block the blood vessels.

The other major category of stroke is known as a hemorrhagic stroke—a stroke that results from hemorrhage or bleeding. This type of stroke occurs when blood vessels bleed into or around the brain. The pressure damages brain tissue. Such bleeding may result from an aneurysm, a balloonlike swelling in the wall of an artery, or from breakage in arteries stressed by long-standing high blood pressure.

Fortunately, unlike high blood pressure, stroke often has warning signals: dizziness; sudden loss of vision; numbness; paralysis in an arm, a leg, or the face; difficulty in speaking; or trouble understanding. An event that causes these symptoms is called a transient ischemic attack, or TIA. Ischemic refers to poor blood supply to an organ or body part. In the case of TIA, the area affected is the brain. A clot may temporarily block a vessel, depriving the brain of blood and the fuel it carries. Because it lasts only a few hours or minutes, people suffering from TIA may be tempted to ignore the symptoms. Ignoring the warning symptoms, experts say, can prove fatal. About a third of those who report TIAs later go on to have complete strokes.

The effects of stroke depend on which brain cells have been damaged, how much damage there has been, how rapidly other areas of brain tissue can take over the work of the damaged cells, and how effectively the body can repair the damaged blood supply system. When one side of the brain is injured, the opposite side of the body is affected. If the stroke hits the right side of the brain, the left limbs can be disabled. In addition, different areas of the brain control different body functions. Since the left side of the brain controls speech and language, someone whose left side is damaged by stroke may develop difficulties in those areas. Sometimes the stroke damages the communication centers in the brain, scrambling messages so that the stroke victim hears sounds but can't decipher what is being said.

Some of the treatment now being proposed includes drugs to inhibit blood clotting. Other researchers are concentrating on the development of new tools to allow

RISK FACTORS FOR STROKE

1. High blood pressure: This is the biggest risk factor, found in 70 percent of hemorrhagic strokes.

2. Heart disease: Coronary artery disease and valve defects can mean blood fails to flow smoothly through the heart, resulting in clots. When these break loose, they can block the brain's supply lines.

3. Diabetes: Diabetes has a destructive effect on blood vessels.

4. Prior stroke.

5. Arteriosclerosis, known to many people as hardening of the arteries. Clumps of fatty substances build up inside the arteries, making their surfaces round and hard. These deposits promote blood clotting.

6. Age: Those over age 55 have increased stroke risk. Men have a greater risk until age 75, then the risk evens out for men and women.

7. Alcohol: Even moderate drinking (two drinks a day) increases the dangers of hypertension and stroke.

8. For women, combining birth control pills and smoking may increase the risk of stroke.

9. Other suspected factors include smoking and obesity.

doctors to see more clearly inside blood vessels. Many experts, however, are convinced the best tool available against stroke is prevention. Here are some suggestions:

• Promptly report any symptoms to your doctor. These include temporary numbness, paralysis, tingling, or weakness in an arm or leg or on one side of the face; temporary blindness; temporary difficulty speaking or understanding speech; loss of strength in a limb; double vision; unexplained headaches; temporary dizziness; and a change in personality or mental ability.

• Have your blood pressure checked regularly. Follow

your doctor's instructions for controlling high blood pressure.

• Avoid foods high in salt, cholesterol, and saturated fat. Emphasize vegetables, fruit, lean meat, fish, skim milk, and skim-milk cheeses. (See Chapter 3.)

• Stop smoking.

• Exercise regularly.

• Avoid alcohol, or drink only in moderation.

Damage to Other Organs   High blood pressure may also cause progressive kidney damage as the narrowing and thickening of the arteries reduce the amount of fluid that the kidney can filter out. The kidney eliminates waste products from the body into the urine. When these products accumulate, the result can be kidney failure.

In addition undetected high blood pressure can damage the lungs, eyes, ears, liver, spleen, and adrenal glands.

THE CHECK-UP

Whether you have symptoms or not, you need to have your blood pressure checked now as a preventive measure. Blood pressure is commonly measured by wrapping an inflatable cuff around the upper arm. Air is pumped into the cuff until circulation is cut off. When a stethoscope is placed below the cuff, there is silence. As the air is slowly let out of the cuff, blood begins to flow again until the heartbeat can be heard through the stethoscope. This is the highest normal pressure (called systolic). The heart should send a column of mercury to a height of about 120 millimeters. At some point, as more and more air is let out of the cuff, the pressure exerted by the cuff decreases so that the sound of the blood pulsing against the artery walls subsides. This is the point of lowest pressure (called diastolic). It normally raises the mercury to about 80 millimeters.

Blood pressure is always expressed in two numbers, which are measurements of millimeters of mercury (mm Hg) or an equivalent.

120 mm Hg.	systolic	(pumping pressure)
80	diastolic	(resting pressure)

Both systolic and diastolic readings are important. The diastolic pressure has traditionally been emphasized because it is less subject to fluctuation. However, recent studies, including the ongoing Framingham heart study, reveal that systolic pressure may be the more significant predictor of a heart attack.

Taking your blood pressure at home is a good idea if you're trying to get your pressure down through diet or drugs and want to monitor it closely. That way you can obtain an accurate picture of blood pressure throughout the day.

If you are taking your blood pressure with a device that does not have a mercury column (the type used in the doctor's office), you should check your machine against a mercury column type at least once a year, since many of the other types are not calibrated or are calibrated inaccurately. Be sure to place the cuff on your arm properly, and make sure the cuff is big enough to encircle your arm without strain. Do not measure your blood pressure in the arm you are using to squeeze the air pressure bulb. Make sure the whole forearm is slightly flexed and supported at heart level on a smooth surface. If you are using a stethoscope or built-in microphone, be sure there are no distracting noises. Be sure, also, that all parts of your machine are in good condition; look for holes in the rubber, dirty valves, or a worn-out cuff. Do not talk while taking your blood pressure.

Blood pressure monitors suitable for home use range from no-frills mechanical gauges—some cost less than

$20—to automated electronic sets that give digital read-outs of pressure and pulse at a price of $45 to $150. The most expensive and automatic units are practically fool-proof. You don the cuff and press a button, and the machine inflates the cuff, "listens" to your pulse, and computes pressure. By contrast, lower-cost mechanical units demand considerable dexterity, good eyesight, and reasonably acute hearing, since you'll have to put on the cuff one-handed, read a dial, and listen with a stetho-scope.

STARTING TREATMENT

If you discover you have high blood pressure, you should start treatment immediately. As with cholesterol levels, opinions on normal blood pressure levels vary. For many years we were taught to add 100 to our age to get our normal systolic reading. The Framingham study told us that no one's systolic pressure should be over 140, nor should the diastolic be allowed to go over 90. The study showed too that both numbers are important.

If you have a reading of 140/90 or above, your physician will want to start lowering your pressure. There are two things he or she can do. One is to start a non-drug treatment, asking you to cut down on salt intake, stop smoking, lose weight, and more. Or he or she may decide to initiate drug therapy by itself or in combination with other methods.

Before you begin treatment, I suggest that you have another reading. Blood pressure can rise while you are in the doctor's office, only to return to normal after the visit. This is called "white coat" or "office" hypertension. One recent New York City study to check the blood pressure of 300 participants in the doctor's office turned up hypertension in 20 percent of the subjects. When these same people were monitored outside the office, only 10 percent had high blood pressure readings.

WHICH TREATMENT TO TRY

Over the past decade a number of methods (including drugs) have been advanced for reducing high blood pressure. Fortunately, even if you have hypertension, it can be controlled under the supervision of a physician. According to a report by the Joint National Committee on Detection, Evaluation, and Treatment of High Blood Pressure, drugs can control hypertension in 80 to 85 percent of all cases, regardless of the initial severity. In some cases blood pressure can be brought down without drugs. Your doctor will help you select the best treatment. Let's look at the most popular.

Behavior Modification
Behavior modification of lifestyle and diet is one of the tools anyone with hypertension should try.

Sodium and Salt   First your doctor will limit your salt intake, since eating excessive amounts of salt probably helped contribute to the trouble. In some genetically susceptible people (those with a family history of hypertension), a relatively high-salt diet from infancy may increase the risk of developing high blood pressure at an older age. Many of us acquired a taste for salt when we were fed baby food with a high sodium content. A Harvard University expedition to the Solomon Islands in the late 1960s and early 1970s showed that blood pressure in eight tribal groups was more closely related to salt than to any other dietary factor. Drs. L. K. Dahl, E. D. Freis, and J. V. Joosens found in separate epidemiological studies in Polynesia, Micronesia, Africa, and South America that people who eat relatively small amounts of salt (five grams or less a day) are remarkably free from hypertension. Conversely, populations that consume large amounts of salt—northern Japanese farmers, for example—have a high incidence of hypertension.

It is impossible to eliminate sodium from your diet, as sodium is an essential mineral for good health. There must be a balance of sodium and water in your body fluids and tissues at all times. Sodium is also essential to maintain normal blood volume, blood pressure, and nerve and muscle function. But the amount of sodium required is so minute—about 220 milligrams, or 1/10th of a teaspoon of salt per day—that most people consume enough without getting near a salt shaker. In fact, because most foods contain salt, it is nearly impossible to limit daily sodium intake to 220 milligrams.

Ordinary salt itself is sodium chloride—40 percent sodium by weight. Amounts are spoken of in terms of grams and milligrams. There are about 28 grams in one ounce and 5.5 grams in a teaspoon. The American Heart Association recommends that individuals limit their salt intake to between 1,000 and 3,000 milligrams a day (about one teaspoon of salt).

Unfortunately, most of us use much more. The average American daily consumes 4,000 to 5,000 milligrams of sodium, or two to three times the recommended amount.

Fortunately, cutting salt intake isn't as difficult as you might think. You can retrain your taste buds to prefer a less salty taste by cutting back on salt a little at a time and by making low-salt substitutions for high-sodium foods. Start by decreasing your intake of processed foods that are loaded with salt: canned soups, bouillon, lunch meats, fast food, and salted snacks—pretzels, potato chips.

I have also found that there is salt in most breakfast cereals, canned fruits, imitation bacon bits, frozen foods, ketchup, and mustard. A six-ounce glass of tomato juice, usually considered a healthy drink, has 450 to 600 milligrams of salt; a fast-food hamburger washed down with a milk shake adds another 300–350 milligrams.

HOW MUCH SODIUM?

Health Factors	Sodium Level	Dietary Guidelines
Healthy person	Sodium is a chemical important to life. It maintains blood volume and pressure by attracting and holding water in the blood vessels. However, we only need 3,000 milligrams per day or less. Most Americans take in much more.	Do not use table salt. A teaspoon of salt contains about 2 grams of sodium (2,000 mg.).
Mild hypertension Mild heart disease Mild fluid retention	1,100–2,000 milligrams per day, preferably less. Follow the advice of your physician if you are on a restricted diet.	Do not use table salt. Use substitutes such as lemon juice, vinegar, homemade relish. Add spices and herbs like onion or garlic powder for zest. (Do not use onion or garlic salt.)
Moderate to severe hypertension Kidney disease Moderate to severe heart disease	1,000–2,000 milligrams per day, preferably less. Follow the advice of your physician if you are on a restricted diet.	Do not use table salt. Look for foods with 140 milligrams or less per serving. Some ingredients that contain sodium are: salt, soy sauce, monosodium glutamate, and baking soda.

HIGH AND LOW SODIUM FOODS

Food Group	Foods to Avoid as Much as Possible	Foods to Look for Instead
Dairy	Buttermilk, processed cheeses, ice cream, milk desserts, butter	Unsalted margarine, skim or lowfat milk, lowfat yogurt, lowfat and low-sodium cheeses *Example:* 4 oz. regular cottage cheese has 455 mg. of sodium 4 oz. dry curd cottage cheese has 15 mg. of sodium
Meat	Canned, salted, smoked meats and fish, oil-packed tuna, canned crabmeat, cold cuts, frankfurters, corned beef, canned hash or stew	Fresh meats, poultry, and fish *Example:* 3 oz. canned shrimp has 1,955 mg. of sodium 3 oz. fresh shrimp has 135 mg. of sodium 3 oz. frozen, prebasted turkey has 355 mg. of sodium 3 oz. fresh turkey has 65 mg. of sodium
Vegetables	Canned vegetables and juices, canned soups, pickles, olives, and sauerkraut	Fresh frozen or low-sodium canned vegetable juices, soups with reduced salt content *Example:* 1 cup canned spinach has 484 mg. sodium 1 cup fresh spinach has 39 mg. of sodium

Food Group	Foods to Avoid as Much as Possible	Foods to Look for Instead
Grain products	Pancake mixes, stuffing mixes, salted crackers, pizza, most dry cereals, baked goods prepared with salt, baking soda, or baking powder	whole-grain, low-salt crackers, breads and cereals with low salt content indicated on labels *Example:* 2 saltine crackers have 70 mg. sodium 2 low-sodium crackers have 2 mg. sodium
Snacks	Pretzels, potato, corn and other chips, salted nuts and snack mixes	Unsalted popcorn, fresh or dried fruit *Example:* 1 cup popcorn popped in oil and salt has 175 mg. sodium 1 cup air-popped popcorn has 1 mg. sodium
Other	Mustard, soy sauce, MSG, catsup, bouillon cubes, salad dressings, meat sauces, many antacid medications, fast-food meals, baking soda, baking powder, self-rising flour, meat tenderizers	Cook meals with little or no salt. Be label smart. Choose foods that show low sodium content. Use low-sodium herbs and spices to add flavor. *Example:* 1 tsp. garlic salt has 1,850 mg. sodium 1 tsp. garlic powder has 1 mg. sodium

One teaspoon of salt contains about 2,000 mg. of sodium. The National Research Council indicates that a safe and adequate sodium intake per day is about 1,100–3,300 mg. for an adult. Estimates place actual sodium consumption by adults at 2,300–6,800 mg. per day.

There are also other invisible culprits, various types of sodium compounds that are added to foods for preservation or to enhance taste. The more common include monosodium glutamate (MSG), sodium bicarbonate (baking soda), sodium nitrate or nitrite (a meat preservative), and baking powder. Sodium also occurs naturally in some drinking water and in water softeners.

Sometimes I find that sodium pops up where least expected. Recently my wife and I took a course in Chinese cooking because we thought it would be fun to be able to cook our favorite foods. We were astonished to find that a highly salted soy sauce and a dab or two of monosodium glutamate were added to practically every recipe. We often hear people comment, "Funny thing about Chinese food—half an hour after I eat I'm hungry again." It's not so funny that after such a meal many complain of a severe headache or other discomfort attributed to monosodium glutamate and referred to in medical journals as "the Chinese restaurant syndrome." Now, since my favorite at a restaurant is Oriental food, I always ask that it be prepared without monosodium glutamate. When I cook it myself, I use lightly salted soy sauce.

To cut down on sodium in your diet, follow these rules:

• Empty the salt shaker, and refill it with herbs or low-sodium seasoning.

• Substitute vinegar or lemon juice for high-salt seasonings.

• Reduce or eliminate salt in recipes. If you simply use half the amount called for, you'll reduce the sodium in your diet without sacrificing taste.

• Read labels for sodium content. Switch to low-sodium products that contain 140 milligrams of sodium or less per serving.

• Drain and rinse processed foods. A one-minute rinse washes away three-fourths of the sodium from canned tuna and nearly half the sodium from canned vegetables.

• Taste food before salting it. Then add less than you normally would, reducing your use of salt gradually until you find yourself adding little or none.

• Use salt-free flavoring substitutes such as garlic and onion powder, paprika, curry, dill, and lemon juice.

READING FOOD LABELS

Be Sodium Smart: Food products can give you information on sodium content in several ways. Your most accurate information on sodium comes from products that post this information. By law, the nutrition information must include the amount of sodium per serving. The amount of sodium will be stated in milligrams per day. There are 1,000 milligrams in a gram.

Sodium descriptions: the food companies describe the amount of sodium in their products in several ways.

Sodium free: these products contain less than 5 milligrams of sodium per serving.

Very low sodium: these products contain 35 milligrams or less per serving.

Reduced sodium: these food products have been reformulated to contain at least 75 percent less sodium than the original product. The label must inform you of the sodium content per serving of the new product and the one it replaces.

Ingredients list: the simplest way to tell whether a store-bought food has a high amount of sodium is to note where the sodium appears on the ingredients list. It it is first, or near the top, the level is relatively high. Many foods that don't taste particularly salty are quite high in sodium. Antacids, dessert products, and most commercially prepared or packaged foods are loaded with sodium. Look for various sodium terms: salt, brine, MSG (monosodium glutamate).

Potassium/Calcium/Magnesium   Potassium, like sodium, is essential for life. Most researchers believe that potassium may both lower blood pressure and help prevent stroke.

"Actually you get tremendous protection from the potassium obtained from eating vegetables and fruits," reports Dr. Louis Tobian of the University of Minnesota. "A single helping of fruits or vegetables daily might cut the risk of stroke as much as 40 percent over an extended period." Tobian and his colleague, Tokuichiro Sugimoto, showed in stroke-prone rats that high blood pressure damages the endothelium, a single layer of cells lining arteries in both rats and humans. That damage can lead to obstruction or rupture of arteries. They also showed that the damage can be almost completely eliminated if rats with high blood pressure are given diets rich in potassium.

"Since the advent of the modern junk-food era," Tobian said, "American diets have been low in potassium, and I am worried about the young singles or marrieds so involved in their careers that they just pick up one junk food after another. I think there is going to be a price paid down the line." Tobian also noted that some studies have shown that bachelors die earlier than married men—and he asserts that a possible explanation could be poor diets and low potassium. People who take diuretics may also need additional potassium, because diuretics can lower the potassium level in the body.

Most fruits and vegetables are good sources of potassium. Among the best are bananas, oranges, grapefruit, strawberries, and potatoes.

A calcium deficiency may also be related to hypertension. Studies show that persons with high blood pressure have less calcium in their diets than persons with normal blood pressure. A study by David McCarron, M.D., and his colleagues examined data from 10,372 people aged 18 to 74 without a history of hypertension. The McCarron analysis revealed a significant inverse correlation between calcium consumption and systolic blood pressure, and other studies now suggest that calcium supplementation may lower high blood pressure in some patients.

Most nutrition experts now recommend that the daily allowance of calcium for women be set at between 1,000 and 1,500 milligrams and at 800 milligrams for men. The daily calcium intake of many women, especially older women, is well below recommended levels. Researchers recommend that most individuals should meet their daily calcium requirements with skim milk, low-fat yogurt, and cottage cheese.

Magnesium also helps reduce high blood pressure, although the exact relationship between magnesium and blood pressure is not fully understood.

Diet Changes   Norman Kaplan, a nationally known hypertension researcher at the University of Texas Southwestern Medical School, Dallas, believes that while some people must use drugs to lower blood pressure, others can do it through diet. Here is what he recommends:

• Use polyunsaturated vegetable margarines and oils in place of butter or hydrogenated oils.

• Enjoy fish, skinless poultry, and veal. Bypass bacon, sausage, ham, lunch meats, and hot dogs—all have added sodium.

• Replace whole-milk-based dairy products with low-fat and nonfat dairy products.

• Eat fresh foods, fresh or frozen vegetables, and fresh or frozen fruits and juices. All have less sodium than processed foods.

- Select a high-fiber diet low in overall fat and rich in whole-grain breads, cereals, fruits, and vegetables.
- Avoid salted nuts, chips, olives, and pickles.

Alcohol and Caffeine   A 1986 Kaiser Permanente report indicated that alcohol in any amount contributes to a rise in blood pressure, independent of coffee or tea consumption, cigarette smoking, body weight, sex, race, or age. Australian researchers have reported that men with high blood pressure can lower blood pressure readings by simply cutting beer consumption to one regular beer a day or by switching to low-alcohol beer. The recommendation here is simply to drink wine, beer, and hard liquor in moderate amounts if you drink at all.

Research on caffeine consumption, while sparse, shows that the caffeine in two cups of coffee can cause a slight rise in blood pressure. In a recent study of male graduates of Johns Hopkins Medical School, Thomas A. Pearson, M.D., Andrea La Croix, Ph.D., and their colleagues found that the more coffee the men regularly drank, the higher the incidence of heart disease. At greatest risk were those who drank at least five cups a day—their rate of cardiac disease was two and a half times the rate for men who did not drink coffee. Enough questions continue to be raised about coffee and cardiovascular health, including blood pressure, to warrant cutting back to below two cups a day.

Unfortunately, decaffeinated coffee may not be a good substitute. Studies by Dr. J. Robert Superka, director of the Lipid Research Clinic at Stanford University, reported that the LDL cholesterol levels of 181 middle-aged men who switched to decaffeinated coffee rose an average of 7 percent, increasing heart attack risk an estimated 12 percent. More research is needed to determine the exact reason for this.

Anger   Since the 1930s researchers have suggested a link between suppressed anger and hypertension. Recent studies seem to confirm that suppressed hostility may have as great an effect on blood pressure as other, more commonly acknowledged risk factors. Anger may be apparent as mild irritation, hostility, or intense aggressiveness. It most often results from blaming others—whether consciously or unconsciously—for one's own mistakes. A study by researchers at the University of Michigan reported that blood pressure was highest among those who resolve anger by repressing it, next highest among those who explode with it, and lowest among those people who discuss their resentment. See Chapter 6 for more about stress and ways to cope with it for the good of your heart.

Weight Loss

Another way of controlling high blood pressure is through weight loss. Numerous studies have shown a connection in both children and adults between being overweight and having high blood pressure. The relationship seems strongest in women, in people with a family history of hypertension, and in those under 60 years of age. Anyone who is both hypertensive and overweight should immediately begin a weight reduction program under a doctor's supervision.

Exercise

Many physicians now believe that it is possible to lower high blood pressure a moderate amount through regular physical activity. Kenneth Cooper and associates at the Cooper Clinic in Dallas found in a study of 3,000 men that there was a difference of four to eight points in blood pressure between separate groups of men and women who were in excellent physical shape and similar groups of men and women in poor physical shape.

Researchers at the University of Wisconsin, Madison, decided to find out which had more effect on blood pressure—rest or exercise. Participants did aerobic exercises (swimming, riding a stationary bike, jogging) for 40 minutes on one day and rested for 40 minutes the next. The investigators then monitored the blood pressures of the participants and administered tests for determining anxiety levels. Both aerobic exercise and relaxation, they discovered, decreased resting blood pressures. Relaxation reduced blood pressure for about 20 minutes. In comparison, aerobic exercise lowered participants' blood pressures and anxiety levels for an average of two to three hours.

Finally, a recently reported study of 14,988 male Harvard alumni found that the incidence of hypertension among the subjects who stayed on an exercise program of vigorous sports activity for at least two hours per week was 30 percent lower than for those who were sedentary. The same was true for subjects who expended 2,000 kilocalories (kcal) per week in leisure-time activities (walking one block or climbing 20 stairs equals about 8 kcal, light sports expend about 5 kcal per minute, and vigorous sports use up around 10 kcal per minute.

Generally exercise is always recommended for people with hypertension (after, of course, they have been examined by a physician). When Walter Mondale was being treated by White House physicians for slightly elevated blood pressure, the physicians recommended that he allow more time for physical exercise. Most doctors tell me they get good results when they put patients with high blood pressure on a program of light jogging, walking, or swimming. (See Chapter 2.)

Drug Therapy
Some physicians prescribe diet and lifestyle modification first. Others ask you to begin a combination of hypertensive drug therapy and lifestyle treatment simultaneously. If possible, I would try to persuade your

DRUGS USED IN TREATING HIGH BLOOD PRESSURE

Drug Class	How They Work	Possible Complications
Diuretic	Rids the body of excess fluid, reducing blood volume and pressure	Impotence, lightheadedness, upset stomach
Beta blocker	Curbs nerve impulses to the heart and blood vessels causing the heart rate to decrease and the blood vessels to relax	Impotence, dizziness, drowsiness, nausea, depression, constipation, decreased heart rate
ACE inhibitor	Prevents the formation of a hormone that increases blood pressure	Itchy rashes, loss of taste or change in taste sensation, abnormal heart rhythms
Calcium antagonist	Reduces pressure on blood vessels by forcing them to relax	Constipation, headache, nausea, fatigue, dizziness

Scene Sutter Hospital Publication Spring 1987

doctor to let you try to lower your blood pressure without drugs first.

There are four types of drugs physicians generally prescribe for high blood pressure: diuretics, beta blockers, calcium antagonists, and ACE (angiotensin-converting enzyme) inhibitors. Each drug works differently. And patients may have to try several before they find one that works best for them. Calcium antagonists and ACE inhibitors, while more expensive than beta blockers and diuretics, have fewer side effects. The factors to consider when selecting a hypertensive drug are age, sex, and race. For example, studies show that blacks and the elderly often respond better to diuretics and calcium antagonists than to beta blockers or ACE inhibitors.

In the 1970s the cost of hypertensive drugs was seldom a barrier to controlling high blood pressure. In the 1990s the cost of medication will become a growing problem.

Once blood pressure has been controlled with medications for at least a year, drug dosage can often be reduced without causing a rise in pressure.

Biofeedback Techniques

Biofeedback is a technique that allows you to monitor your blood pressure (as well as other functions) in order to alter it. In biofeedback training you are attached to an electrical instrument that signals high blood pressure by beeping or flashing. This feedback information then allows you to gain control over your blood pressure.

To find a biofeedback practitioner, enquire at a local medical center or university, or write to the Biofeedback Certification Institute of America, 4301 Owens Street, Wheat Ridge, Colorado 80033, to order their directory of practitioners qualified to treat hypertension.

Relaxation Exercises

Daily relaxation, including a number of types of meditation, has proved effective in reducing high blood pressure. Taking time to relax deeply for 15 to 20 minutes at least once, but preferably twice, a day is recommended for blood pressure control.

Deep Breathing   Slow, deep breathing helps promote relaxation. Place one hand over your stomach and the other on your upper chest. Notice which hand moves as you breathe. Allow your stomach to rise as you breathe slowly in while keeping your upper chest still. This deep-breathing technique allows you to fill the bottom of your lungs as if you were filling a balloon. Continue to breathe with your abdomen. Slow in-breath, slow out-breath. Allow your mind to think only about the breathing rhythm. Continue for 10 to 20 minutes. Notice how relaxed you feel.

Mental Relaxation/Meditation   Meditation is thinking about one thing only. An effective technique for reducing blood pressure was explained by Dr. Herbert Benson in his book *The Relaxation Response.*

Begin by deep breathing, allowing your mind to think only about your breathing. Then think the word *one* each time you breathe out. Breathe slowly in, and as you breathe out, think "one." If other thoughts come into your mind, notice them objectively, then go back to noticing your breathing and think "one" as you breathe out. Continue this for 10 to 15 minutes or as desired.

Mini-Relaxations   A mini-relaxation is a very short relaxation technique that can be performed for a few seconds or minutes. Here are two to try.

Mini-relaxation 1: Anytime throughout the day, notice how your muscles feel. If you feel tension or muscle tightness anywhere, start deep abdominal breathing. As you take a deep breath in, imagine you can relax the tight muscle. As you breathe out, feel the muscle become loose, limp, and relaxed.

Mini-relaxation 2: Anytime, start breathing deeply. Take a slow deep breath in. As you breathe out, let your shoulders become limp, your forehead smooth, and your face soft. Then imagine your arms and legs becoming heavier and warmer. Imagine you are sitting in the sun. Continue deep breathing for awhile. Remain awake, alert, and relaxed.

Leaving hypertension untreated is like playing Russian roulette. The time between its onset and the death of the hypertensive patient has been estimated at about

20 years. For the first two-thirds of this time, it is likely that no symptoms will be experienced. After that, vital organs begin to fail. Untreated, the victim survives an average of six more years. A stroke often occurs just when a person is starting to relax after struggling all his or her life.

A close relative of mine is a typical victim. A brilliant man, he graduated at the top of his class from a major university and worked all his life as a manager in a big corporation. Shortly after his retirement, he had a stroke that seriously affected his mental capacities. Recently I visited him at the rest home where he was confined. In one of his lucid moments, he looked out the window and said, "Please, God, I don't know what is the matter with me, but I know I'm not my former self. Please make me like I used to be."

With cases like these, there is little doubt that hypertension needs to be brought under control and kept that way throughout your life. In the next chapter we will cover smoking—an additional factor that causes increased blood pressure and cardiac disease.

5
A Smoke-Free Life

Ask any physician what you can do to prevent cardiovascular disease, and the first thing most will tell you is, "Stop smoking!" The reason? Tobacco smoke is more deadly as a risk factor for heart disease than all the others combined! Indeed, this year 1 out of 6 deaths will occur as a direct result of a smoking-caused disease: lung cancer, coronary heart disease, and emphysema, a disease that gradually destroys breathing capacity. Of those who now smoke, 1 out of 2 will die prematurely.

Currently smoking is blamed for 25 percent of all coronary heart disease, 30 percent of all cancer deaths, and 80 percent of all bronchitis and emphysema. Half of all strokes of people under age 65 stem from smoking. The American Heart Association estimates that this year more than 350,000 Americans will die from smoking-related heart disease. These are deaths that could be avoided if everyone gave up cigarettes.

As Dr. William Bennett, associate editor of the *Harvard Medical Letter*, states, "At any age, smoking increases the probability of dying [early] by 70 percent, while smoking two packs a day increases the probability by 100 percent."

In 1980 Dr. C. C. Seltzer of Harvard University reported a statistical association between cigarette smoking and coronary heart disease. Dr. Peter H. Levine of the Tufts–New England Medical Center found that smoking even one standard filter-tipped cigarette had a marked effect on the clogging of the arteries. When researchers looked at several risk factors in combination with smoking, the results were dramatic. Smokers with high blood pressure are 22.2 times as likely to develop coronary artery disease as nonsmokers without hypertension. Smokers with high cholesterol have 18.9 times as much risk as nonsmokers, and smokers with diabetes have 22.3 times as much.

Traditionally women have lived longer than men. Unfortunately, this advantage may soon be reduced in the United States. It all depends on women's smoking habits. If women continue smoking more, as studies show they are, their incidence of lung cancer and heart problems could climb high enough to turn the entire picture around.

According to Dr. G. H. Miller, director of studies on smoking at Edinboro State College, Edinboro, Pennsylvania, women are more prone to the ravages of smoking than men. Until now, he says, they have lived longer to some extent because they have smoked much less than men. But this is changing. And the countdown reversing their eight-year longevity advantage could begin in approximately 5 to 15 years, so that somewhere in the first half of the 21st century it may be men who are outliving women.

Twenty years ago males accounted for most smoking-related complications. At that time men had nine times as many reported cases of emphysema as did women. Today the ratio is 5 men to 1 woman.

Besides women's life expectancy, smoking also affects their fertility. Female smokers have more trouble getting pregnant and face a greater risk of spontaneous abortion, stillbirth, and premature delivery. Their babies are smaller at birth and have increased risk of dying in early infancy.

Other dangers to female smokers include a greater risk of postmenopausal osteoporosis, which weakens bone structure and leads to fractures that may result in prolonged disability and death. Lung cancer recently surpassed breast cancer as the leading cause of cancer death in women. Recent evidence also suggests that cancer of the cervix is more common in women who smoke than in nonsmokers.

THE TOXIC CONNECTION

No one knows for sure what elements in cigarette smoke cause cardiac disease, but it is known that cigarette smoke contains at least 3,000 toxic chemicals of all types. And from the Surgeon General's Report we do know that tobacco smoke contains the following: carbon monoxide, carbon dioxide, benzene, toluene, formaldehyde, acetone, hydrogen cyanide, ammonia, nitrogen oxide, formic acid, acetic acid, nicotine, tar, benzopyrene, and other pollutants. The smoke from a single cigarette contains about 100 times the cyanide of the two grapes from Chile that were impounded by the government in March 1989.

Within seconds after a smoker takes a puff (chewing tobacco has the same effects), the cardiovascular system becomes highly stressed. Nicotine in the bloodstream causes several things to happen. The pulse increases 15 to 25 beats per minute, and the blood pressure rises about 10 to 20 points on both the systolic and diastolic readings. What's more, the effects created by smoking one cigarette last as long as two to four hours.

Carbon monoxide and nicotine are thought to be the main threats to the heart in cigarette smoke. Carbon monoxide robs oxygen from the red blood cells. In the average smoker, 16 percent of the red blood cells' oxygen-carrying capacity is taken over by carbon monoxide. Heavy smokers subject themselves to eight times the carbon monoxide exposure allowed in industry.

Nicotine constricts the arteries by 50 percent. This reduction decreases the blood flow to the heart by about one-fourth. Nicotine is also concentrated 3.7 times higher in the heart than in the blood. In people whose arteries have been damaged, this situation is aggravated because their hearts already receive less than the normal amount of oxygen. In addition, nicotine stimulates a heart rate increase of as many as 20 beats a minute, which for most smokers is as much as 20,000 extra beats a day—an increase that lasts for at least 20 minutes after the individual puts out his or her cigarette.

The person who smokes a pack and a half per day gets a yearly radiation dose in all parts of the lungs equal to 300 chest x-rays. Cigarette smoke also contains nitrogen dioxide and hydrogen cyanide, two volatile gases so destructive that they were the primary ingredients used in poison gas during World War I.

Since the lungs are responsible for the intake of oxygen needed by the heart, there is a direct connection between lung health and heart health. If the lungs are damaged by emphysema, the small bronchial tubes become clogged, resulting in extensive destruction of the air sacs, the places where oxygen, carbon dioxide, and other gases are exchanged with the blood. When the air sacs are constricted, an inadequate exchange of air leads to poor oxygenation of the body. This creates a loss of energy and limits the body's capacity to rid the body of the impurities from cigarettes.

THE MYSTERIOUS LINK

It is obvious that cigarette smoking puts a strain on the heart. But just what the exact mechanism is or why it increases heart attack risk is still a mystery. Research at Japan's Kyoto University indicates that cigarette

WHAT SMOKING DOES TO THE HEART

1. *Smoking makes the heart work harder.* Nicotine and other ingredients in cigarette smoke increase blood pressure, the heart rate, and the force of each heartbeat.

2. *Smoking reduces the blood supply to the heart.* Nicotine causes the arteries to constrict. This reduces the flow of blood to the heart muscle.

3. *Smoking releases hormones.* Smoking releases norepinephrine and epinephrine into the bloodstream. This can cause severe spasm in some arteries.

4. *Smoking reduces the blood's oxygen-carrying capacity.* The carbon dioxide released by burning tobacco restricts the ability of the red blood cells to carry oxygen.

5. *Smoking thickens the blood.* Because it has less oxygen-carrying capacity, the blood becomes thicker, making it even more difficult for the heart to pump the blood through constricted arteries.

6. *Smoking damages artery walls.* The toxic by-products of burning tobacco are believed to cause further damage to the artery walls.

---

smoke extract can modify HDLs (the good cholesterol) to decrease their effectiveness.

A study of nearly 10,000 children who smoked showed that all had lower levels of HDL and higher levels of LDL (the lipoprotein believed to deposit cholesterol in the artery walls) than nonsmoking children. According to Dr. John A. Morrison of the Cincinnati Lipid Research Clinic, the 11 percent decrease found in their HDL levels could be a significant risk factor. Since none of these children had been smoking long, these studies may indicate that HDL levels go down dramatically immediately after a person starts to smoke.

Very recent research by the American Health Foundation on 20,000 people in Jackson, Mississippi, and Lansing, Michigan (including a backup study of Hartford, Connecticut, Atlanta, and Miami) found that every cigarette raises the total cholesterol half a point on average. The researchers discovered that the more you smoke, the higher your cholesterol. Exactly how cigarette smoking affects cholesterol levels is not known, but Harris speculates that smoking may alter levels of sex hormones that have an effect on serum cholesterol.

A study of 49 pairs of identical twins in Finland shows the association of smoking with carotid atherosclerosis is highly significant even after statistically adjusting for age, cholesterol level, blood pressure, and other factors. Dr. William Moskowitz of the Medical College of Virginia reports that smoking also increases the thickness of the heart walls and stiffens the aorta, forcing the heart to work harder.

THE HAZARDS OF SECONDHAND SMOKE

Even though you don't smoke, just living or working with smokers may endanger your health. Scientific studies show that exposure to the smoke of others, known as passive or involuntary smoking, may increase your risk of heart disease, emphysema, bronchitis, and stroke.

The smoke that fills the air from a burning cigarette is composed of two types of smoke: the smoke inhaled and exhaled by the smoker—mainstream smoke—and the smoke that comes from a burning cigarette, cigar, or pipe between puffs—sidestream smoke. Unfortunately most of the smoke that reaches the lungs of nonsmokers is sidestream smoke, the more hazardous of the two.

Sidestream smoke has 2.5 times as much carbon monoxide as mainstream smoke. Long-term exposure to sidestream smoke can cause or aggravate heart disease as carbon monoxide narrows blood vessels and combines with hemoglobin to reduce the blood's oxygen-carrying ability.

This effect of carbon monoxide is one reason cigarette

LOVE-YOUR-HEART SMOKING FACTS

These facts are ones that most impressed me as I read numerous publications while researching this book.

Cigarette smokers have 70 percent more heart attacks than nonsmokers.

Smoking and birth control pills increase heart attacks by 39 percent.

One in six deaths in this country is due to smoking.

There are one million deaths a year in industrialized nations from tobacco.

Twenty-five percent of smokers quit successfully on the first try. Over 73 percent are successful by the fourth try.

A recent survey by the American Association of Retired Persons showed that 65 percent of smokers over age 49 would like to quit.

More than 90 percent of all smokers manage to quit without any kind of help.

By reducing circulation of blood to the skin, smoking makes you look older. Wrinkles appear, especially at the corners of the eyes and around the lips and neck.

The nonsmoker enjoys a 23 percent reduction in premiums for term life insurance.

smoking has long been a primary risk factor in coronary heart disease. Recently studies have begun to show a relationship between involuntary smoking and heart disease, reporting an increase in heart disease for passive smokers and suggesting that tobacco smoke speeds the onset of angina in people who have cardiovascular disease.

Even stronger evidence links tobacco smoke exposure to increased risk for cancer. After a thorough analysis of all of the world's epidemiological studies on passive smoking, the National Academy of Science concluded in

1986 that the risk of lung cancer is roughly 30 percent higher for nonsmoking spouses of smokers than for nonsmoking spouses of nonsmokers. Other independent investigations confirm this danger.

Researchers monitored the smoke-filled rooms at a meeting of the American Academy of Allergy and found that nonsmokers' lungs registered four times the normal carbon monoxide level even though they hadn't touched a cigarette. Eight parts per million of carbon monoxide were measured in the lungs of nonsmokers after they had left a room where smoking was permitted, compared to only two parts per million in a room where smoking was banned.

A 1978 study by Dr. Wilbert S. Aronow of the Veterans Administration Hospital in Long Beach, California, found that sitting near cigarette smokers made people with coronary heart problems more susceptible to the sometimes crippling chest pain called angina. When they were exposed to secondhand smoke, their heart rates increased, their blood pressures rose, and three of them died as a result of irregular heartbeats. Explains Dr. Aronow, "While breathing other people's smoke is not as bad as smoking, the passive smoker is still at significant risk."

Children are not immune to the problem. Many children of smokers have more middle-ear and respiratory infections, more hospitalizations for bronchitis and pneumonia, and a smaller rate of increase in lung function than children of parents who do not smoke. Tobacco smoke in the home also increases the incidence of respiratory illnesses such as pneumonia and bronchitis in children, and the effects are enhanced if both parents smoke. In addition, according to the American Heart Association, even low amounts of secondhand smoke affect the heart and blood fats of children. One study reported at the meeting found that secondhand smoke lowered the HDL (good cholesterol) levels of a group of teenage boys and put them at a high risk of accelerated heart disease in later years.

Spouses of smokers too are at high risk. In studying 7,115 women between the ages of 30 and 59, Dr. Michael J. Martin reported to the American Health Association Las Vegas meeting that women married to smokers had 3.4 times as many myocardial infarction heart attacks as the wives of never-smokers, and those married to former smokers had 1.9 times as many myocardial infarctions. In a collaborating study, Dr. Cedric Garland of the University of California in San Diego found that 2.7 times as many wives of current or former smokers developed ischemic heart disease as did wives of never-smokers.

Former surgeon general C. Everett Koop estimates that other people's tobacco smoke causes more death than all other air pollution combined, with the exception of asbestos. Unfortunately, many nonsmokers apparently aren't aware of the danger or don't care.

REGULATIONS

The government cannot regulate smoking that occurs in the home, but public support as well as information on the adverse health effects of exposure to tobacco smoke has helped launch the movement toward work site restrictions. Surveys have found that more than 75 percent of Americans favor restricting smoking to limited areas at the work site. In addition nonsmokers say they would like the air they breathe to be free of the unpleasant odor and irritation of tobacco smoke. In interviews with 13,000 smokers and nonsmokers, more than 70 percent were annoyed at the smoke of others, and almost two-thirds want smoking restricted. The surgeon general has suggested that smoking in the workplace be banned in order to reduce exposure of nonsmokers to tobacco smoke.

There is evidence that progress is being made, since several states and dozens of municipalities have passed legislation regulating smoking in the private workplace. The 1990 Health Objectives for the Nation adopted by the Public Health Service recommend all 50 states pass laws by the early 1990s that prohibit smoking in enclosed public places and that require separate smoking areas at the work site and in restaurants. Private and voluntary efforts have been important here. A majority of the public now supports the right of nonsmokers to breathe smoke-free air, and many private employers have voluntarily put regulations into effect in their own places of business. Recently too, the U.S. Army has issued a worldwide directive prohibiting smoking in any but designated areas.

There is still a long way to go. I still remember observing a cardiologist put out his cigarette as he prepared to give a paper on how to prevent a fatal heart attack. Fortunately this is not typical of younger physicians. A recent study shows that there is a continuous downturn in smoking among first- and second-year medical students.

REVERSING THE EFFECTS

It is impossible to reverse all of the effects of smoking while continuing to smoke, but research conducted at an army medical research laboratory blood bank at Fort Knox, Kentucky, showed that even a few minutes of mild exercise can go a long way toward cleaning the bloodstream of poisons from cigarette smoke.

After giving blood, one group of smokers was asked to perform three to four minutes of mild body exercises, while another group did no exercise. The first group showed a 10 percent decrease in carbon monoxide levels, while the second group showed only a 5 percent decrease—the natural drop due to the passage of gases through the bloodstream.

If you are a smoker, a disciplined exercise program also seems to be the best answer to ridding yourself of the habit. People who begin a fitness program quickly learn that rhythmic endurance exercise and smoking don't mix. Exercise will help relieve irritability, encourage restful sleep, and alleviate depression during nicotine withdrawal.

If you have been sedentary, you should gradually include activity as part of a daily schedule. For a good exercise program, see Chapter 2.

WHEN SHOULD YOU QUIT?

There is a bright side to the relationship between smoking and cardiovascular health. Within 30 minutes after a person stops smoking, the chance of dying from cardiac arrest begins to drop tremendously. After a few days, the nicotine is washed from the system, resulting in a slower pulse, lower blood pressure, and reduced coronary artery spasms. Within a few weeks, the red blood cells carrying carbon monoxide are replaced by new ones carrying oxygen. In fact, in about 120 days, all have been replaced.

No matter how long you have smoked, you can bounce back. A few smoke-free years will put any smoker back in the same health-fitness category as the nonsmoker. Almost immediately you will breathe easier, have more energy with less sleep, digest food with less stomach upset, cough less, and have a lower heart rate.

Research shows that although anyone who smokes has a greater risk of sudden death from heart attack than a nonsmoker, this risk drops sharply within one or two years after quitting.

All research indicates that you are never too old to stop. Seniors in their sixties, seventies, and eighties can reduce their risk of heart attack by giving up cigarettes. A study based on individuals with already clogged arteries found that over a five-year period the death rate among older people who continued to smoke was 70 percent higher than for seniors who gave up smoking. And while the damage from atherosclerosis may have been done, much of the damage from smoking occurs while smoking and is alleviated almost immediately when smoking is stopped . . . regardless of age. After two years of being a nonsmoker, you have a chance of premature death from a heart attack that approaches the risk of someone who has never smoked.

This means that the best thing you can do for your heart health, right now, is to stop smoking.

THE BARRIERS TO QUITTING

There is little doubt that quitting is difficult. During the 1980s about 17.3 million men and women tried for at least a day each year, but only 1.3 million managed to abstain for a year or more. Of those, about 40 percent begin smoking in 2 to 10 years, with only half trying to quit again.

The main problem is that nicotine is addictive, although, unlike other addictive substances, it does not interfere with normal behavior or thinking. Smokers have been found to continue their habit in order to avoid the unpleasantness that comes from stopping: nausea, headaches, constipation, diarrhea, weight gain, and an inability to concentrate.

The inhaling smoker receives nicotine jolts that give a hard-to-define but pleasant feeling. For this reason quitting is not a simple matter. Three out of four smokers who try to kick the habit eventually start to smoke again because of the severity of withdrawal symptoms. A UCLA study, however, discovered that those who quit "cold turkey" are less affected by these symptoms than those who try to quit gradually.

As a rationalization, many people use the excuse that they can't stop smoking because smoking helps keep the weight off. A report in the *Journal of the American Medical Association* does show that cigarette smokers as a group weigh less for their height than nonsmokers and that the cessation of smoking does lead to some weight gain.

However, according to the National Institute on Aging in Baltimore, smokers also have significantly larger waist-hip ratios than nonsmokers. Fat distribution patterns with high waist-hip ratios are associated with risk factors such as abnormal serum lipid levels, high blood pressure, and glucose intolerance, which have been linked to increased risks for coronary heart disease, diabetes, and early death. The study also reports that while smokers who quit smoking gained an average of five pounds, their waist-hip ratios did not increase significantly. On the other hand, former smokers who suffered a relapse and started smoking again experienced a significant increase in waist-hip ratios.

Many young smokers, to avoid giving up smoking altogether, have turned to cigarettes with a reduced tar and nicotine content. Unfortunately, as reported by the surgeon general, there is no such thing as a safe cigarette. Although some cigarettes seem to contribute less to the risk of lung cancer than others, they have not been shown to have less impact on the risk of cardiovascular disease. As the surgeon general pointed out, these "lite" cigarettes may even be more dangerous for pregnant women than for other people. Also, people who turn to these kinds of cigarettes may smoke more and inhale more deeply. In addition, a large number of young people, believing that these cigarettes are safe, have recently taken up smoking. The newer brands with reduced yields of nicotine and carbon monoxide don't seem to offer much hope either. A recent study to evaluate the effect of "low-yield cigarettes" on women concluded that they are extremely toxic and no alternative to quitting.

There also seem to be some problems with the new

WHY DO YOU SMOKE?

Here are some statements made by people to describe what they get out of smoking cigarettes. How often do you feel this way when smoking? Circle one number for each statement. Important: **Answer every question.**

		Always	Frequently	Occasionally	Seldom	Never
A.	I smoke cigarettes in order to keep myself from slowing down.	5	4	3	2	1
B.	Handling a cigarette is part of the enjoyment of smoking it.	5	4	3	2	1
C.	Smoking cigarettes is pleasant and relaxing.	5	4	3	2	1
D.	I light up a cigarette when I feel angry about something.	5	4	3	2	1
E.	When I have run out of cigarettes I find it almost unbearable until I can get them.	5	4	3	2	1
F.	I smoke cigarettes automatically without even being aware of it.	5	4	3	2	1
G.	I smoke cigarettes to stimulate me, to perk myself up.	5	4	3	2	1
H.	Part of the enjoyment of smoking a cigarette comes from the steps I take to light up.	5	4	3	2	1
I.	I find cigarettes pleasurable.	5	4	3	2	1

J.	When I feel uncomfortable or upset about something, I light up a cigarette.	5	4	3	2	1
K.	I am very much aware of the fact when I am not smoking a cigarette.	5	4	3	2	1
L.	I light up a cigarette without realizing I still have one burning in the ashtray.	5	4	3	2	1
M.	I smoke cigarettes to give me a "lift."	5	4	3	2	1
N.	When I smoke a cigarette, part of the enjoyment is watching the smoke as I exhale it.	5	4	3	2	1
O.	I want a cigarette most when I am comfortable and relaxed.	5	4	3	2	1
P.	When I feel "blue" or want to take my mind off cares and worries, I smoke cigarettes.	5	4	3	2	1
Q.	I get a real gnawing hunger for a cigarette when I haven't smoked for a while.	5	4	3	2	1
R.	I've found a cigarette in my mouth and didn't remember putting it there.	5	4	3	2	1

Scores can vary from 3 to 15. Any score 11 and above is high; any score 7 and below is low.

smokeless cigarette. The new cigarette has no cancer-causing tars, produces almost none of the smoke that irritates nonsmokers, and doesn't create an ash because the tobacco in it doesn't burn. However, this cigarette does deliver a substantial dose of nicotine, acting as a "delivery system" for this addictive drug. Tests now show that when you draw air past this new cigarette's smoldering charcoal tip through a cylinder packed with nicotine, tobacco, and flavoring agents, you can achieve blood levels of nicotine nearly as high as from smoking an ordinary cigarette. You also inhale a significant amount of carbon monoxide, which, as already explained, has been implicated as a further cause of heart disease.

HOW TO QUIT SMOKING

Although quitting "cold turkey" is the ideal way to stop smoking, many people find they just cannot quit all at once. Quitting smoking can be a process. It doesn't have to happen all at once. Smokers try, try, and try again—an average of three times before they finally quit.

To stop smoking, you must start thinking and acting like a nonsmoker and begin to learn new ways of relaxing, coping with stress, cutting the appetite, and dealing with boredom instead of reaching for a cigarette. For many smokers this process takes time.

To stop smoking, you must really want to quit. For some people the daily coughing, shortness of breath, and decreased ability to perform physical activity provide the motivation. For others the embarrassment of smoking around nonsmokers who disapprove is enough. For still others the deciding factor is the risk of lung cancer and heart disease.

Consultants say that once you make the decision to stop smoking you should pick a "Target Quit Day." This is a day when you will attempt to put aside cigarettes forever. During the preparation stage, you may want to change your smoking habits to make it easier to stop. This could mean switching brands, cutting back a little each day, and postponing the urge to smoke. Some smokers accumulate ashes and butts in a jar so that they begin to look at the distasteful aspect of smoking. At this stage it may help to start watching nonsmokers to see how they handle the stress and boredom that usually follow any attempt to kick the habit.

If you have a relapse, don't assume that you have gone back to your old habits. Simply set up a new Target Quit Day and start again.

Now here are some methods to try.

SELF-HELP

Ninety percent of smokers who quit do so without the help of a formal program or smoking device. If you choose to quit on your own, numerous pamphlets and self-help materials are available from the American Heart Association, the American Lung Association, and the American Cancer Society, as well as from your physician's office. You need to be highly motivated to stick with the informal programs. Light smokers not heavily dependent on nicotine will do best with a self-help approach.

1. Get rid of all your cigarettes, lighters, matches, and ashtrays. Clean all ashtrays in your car. Brush your teeth and rinse your mouth thoroughly to get rid of smoker's breath.

2. Pick a time when you are not involved in a stressful situation either at home or at work.

3. Set a date, then quit "cold turkey." (This is what worked for most reformed smokers.) Share this date with your friends, family, and coworkers. Ask for support.

4. Spend some time in environments that don't allow smoking: the nonsmoking section of a restaurant, a library, and similar places.

5. Take deep breaths whenever you have the urge to smoke. Hold your breath for several seconds, then release it slowly. This exercise simulates smoking . . . except the air you inhale is clean.

6. If the nicotine habit is linked to your smoking, ask your doctor about nicotine gum.

7. Walk, swim, or jog.

8. If your habit is linked with another habit, change both. If you love to smoke and drink coffee, switch to tea or to lemon with water. If you smoke in your car, open the windows. If you smoke when on the phone, stand up to make yourself uncomfortable.

9. Put money in a jar with other friends who are quitting. Add more money each month. In 12 months, the nonsmokers divide the pot.

10. Associate cigarette smoking with a negative image: a fat person with a cigarette dangling from his or her lips, a picture of the lungs of a three-pack-a-day smoker who died of lung cancer, the clogged arteries of a smoker.

11. Visualize your worst smoking image: the time you burned a hole in your best suit, the time you started a fire. Visualize Sammy Davis, Jr., Arthur Godfrey, Ed Murrow, and Yul Brynner, who were all heavy smokers and who all died of lung cancer.

12. Use oral substitutes: sugarless gum, lemon drops, peanuts, carrot sticks. Avoid spicy foods and foods with sugar—they trigger the desire to smoke.

13. Don't use weight gain as an excuse. Most people gain only a few pounds when they quit. The truth is that you would have to add *125 pounds* before you

suffered the same heart damage as that created by smoking one pack of cigarettes a day.

14. Take it one urge at a time. It is easier to say no for a few minutes than to say you have quit forever. Don't think about tomorrow or the days to come. Just get through today.

Group Support

Group stop-smoking programs are offered through the American Lung Association and the American Cancer Society, at hospitals, and through many employers. These group programs combine behavior modification methods and education to give the smoker skills that will help him or her function without cigarettes. The support group is important in helping the smoker get through the early stages. The group approach is also fairly effective for the smoker who has tried self-help techniques and needs more support.

Nicotine Gum

Doctor-prescribed nicotine gum is a way of providing the smoker with nicotine without the gases and chemicals. Nicotine gum is the only form of nicotine replacement that is approved for use by the Food and Drug Administration. Nicotine patches, nicotine spray, and drugs for curbing withdrawal symptoms are not approved for use in stopping smoking.

This method is useful for smokers who are heavily dependent on nicotine or who have trouble with the withdrawal symptoms. Sometimes nicotine gum is combined with a group support program to help attack the problem in several ways.

Hypnosis and Acupuncture

Some individuals succeed with the help of acupuncture and hypnosis. These treatment techniques help increase motivation, but for many smokers the effects don't last very long. Acupuncture and hypnosis, however, are useful for getting through the first several weeks of any attempt to stop smoking.

WHEN YOU FIRST QUIT

On the first few days without cigarettes, everything seems unfamiliar. This feeling reaches its peak within 48 to 72 hours after quitting. The main problem is nicotine withdrawal. After several years of smoking, the body gets used to a certain nicotine level. When stopping smoking, people often experience body or mood changes. As the body adjusts to the absence of nicotine, the following symptoms may appear:

• Sluggishness/tiredness: Since there is no longer a nicotine stimulant in the bloodstream, the first reaction is some sluggishness.

• Irritability/nervousness: Many individuals get extremely restless and nervous. Often there is sleeplessness or night restlessness. Sometimes they tend to snap at other people. This initial reaction may be alleviated by exercise.

• Dry mouth/cough: Often individuals who quit smoking experience a dry cough, since the body is ridding the lungs of mucus. Since not as much new mucus is produced, the mouth may become dry.

• Hunger: Sometimes people who stop smoking will experience intense hunger pains for the first few weeks. Often you can alleviate this by drinking a glass of water.

Here are some tips to help you through this period:

1. Lower your caloric intake before you quit smoking.
2. If you crave sweets, try raw fruits and vegetables or sugar-sweet substitutes instead of candy and cookies.

3. If you need something to suck on, try sugar-free gum or sugar-free hard candy.

4. Reduce portion sizes at mealtimes.

5. Reduce the fatty foods in your diet—substitute fruits and vegetables.

6. Keep fatty snack foods such as potato chips out of sight. Substitute low-calorie snacks.

7. Rely on aerobic exercise to burn calories.

It is important to understand that the initial symptoms are temporary. During this stage it is helpful to practice deep-breathing exercises and relaxation and to begin breaking associations with cigarettes. Always focus on the immediate benefits of quitting—less frequent cough, lower heart rate, the better taste of food, improved sense of smell, and a sense of being in control.

After the initial one to two weeks of abstinence, ex-smokers must get serious about incorporating some permanent changes in their lives. This is the time to replace cigarettes with other ways to manage stress, emotions, weight control, boredom, even loneliness. Activities such as physical exercise, gardening, playing a musical instrument, finding a new hobby, or joining social groups will help.

Some people are now talking about legislation to make possession of cigarettes illegal. Obviously something as radical as this is not going to happen, at least not in the near future. And even modest antismoking legislation is difficult to pass. In the meantime, however, our hearts can't wait for legislation to make the decision for us. Smoking is one risk factor in heart disease over which we have control. Since we can all choose whether to smoke or not, it seems foolish to continue this dangerous habit. If you want to bypass a bypass, you can start now, by deciding not to smoke.

6
Handling Stress
and Distress

. . . It's not the large things that
send a man to the
madhouse . . . no, it's the
    continuing series of
small tragedies
that send a man to the madhouse
        . . .
not the death of his love
but a shoelace that snaps
with no time left . . .

—Charles Bukowski

Although heart disease is widely referred to as America's number one killer, the real culprit is the individual's unhealthy reaction to stress. Experts agree that overreacting to daily stress, when combined with poor eating habits and lack of exercise, can deal the final blow to the body's autoimmune and other life-preserving systems. As a result, stress can well be considered the number one public health threat of the 1990s.

According to one survey, during any six-month period approximately 29 million Americans, or 18 percent of the population, will have a stress-related alcohol, drug abuse, or mental health disorder. Over 57 million Americans suffer from stress-related hypertension. Over the last several years, over $13 billion has been spent per year on medical care for stress-related stroke victims. And more than one in four Americans suffer from some form of stress-related cardiovascular disease.

STRESS IS INEVITABLE

In a now-famous study, University of Washington psychiatrist Thomas Holmes determined that the single common denominator for all types of stress is change in an individual's life pattern. This means that any change in your regular pattern of living—including taking a vacation, divorce, getting a raise, the death of a spouse, buying a house, and even Christmas—creates stress, which may be positive or negative. Any out-of-the-ordinary event creates stress.

In an attempt to measure the impact of life-changing events, Holmes and psychologist Richard Rahe asked 5,000 people to rate the amount of social readjustment required for various events. The result is the widely used Holmes-Rahe scale. Here is a sample of what they found:

Life Event	Stress Points
Death of spouse	100
Marriage	50
Divorce	73
Pregnancy	40
Marital separation	65
Buying a house	31
Imprisonment	63
Christmas	12

Holmes showed that in a sample of 88 young doctors, those who had a total life-stress rating of 300 or more units had a 70 percent chance of suffering ulcers, psychiatric disturbances, cancer, heart attacks, broken bones, and similar difficulties within a year. Those who scored under 200 had only a 37 percent incidence of health problems within a year. Over the years this scale has proved to be a good predictor of individuals who would suffer future stress. This scale has proved so reliable that by tallying up the life-stress points of healthy football players, Holmes and Rahe were able to predict which ones would be injured during the next season.

THE NECESSITY FOR STRESS

We have come to view all stress as harmful. The truth is, it isn't. Dr. Hans Selye, director of the Institute of Experimental Medicine and Surgery at the University of Montreal, defined stress as

> the nonspecific response of our body to any demand made on it. It is immaterial whether the agent or situation we face is pleasant or unpleasant; all that counts is the intensity of the demand for readjustment or adaption.
>
> For instance, the mother who is told her son died in battle suffers a terrible mental shock. If years later, it turns out the news was false and the son unexpectedly walks into her room alive, she experiences extreme joy. The results of the two events, sorrow and joy, are opposite, but the stress they produce may well be the same.

The truth is that when someone says he or she is under stress, that person means excessive stress or distress. There is a great deal of evidence to indicate that every individual needs some stress for happiness. There are many individual differences, but stress is really the spice of life. As Dr. Selye said at a 1973 meeting of the Million Dollar Round Table of Life Insurance Executives, "Not only is stress unavoidable, it is undesirable to avoid it. Any demand on the body causes stress, and stress is a great stimulus to achievement. You shouldn't try to avoid it, you should try to enjoy it."

Playing tennis and struggling against an opponent puts you as an individual under stress. So does mowing the lawn, trying to make a big sale, or struggling to get an *A* on a test. Yet most of us thrive on this kind of stress. Many people take great joy in winning a game, taking part in a contest, or trying to build a business.

We could avoid stress by doing nothing, but it would create a joyless world. Imagine living in the same room all your life. You wouldn't be bothered by stress, but you would wither away from boredom. Stress itself is not really harmful, since it helps us live life to the fullest.

STRESS/DISTRESS

Stress, of course, can stem from simple or extremely complicated events. You might, for instance, put yourself under stress by accidentally writing a check without funds to cover it. You handle it, however, by transferring funds from your savings account.

Another example might be the theft of your wallet, containing cash and credit cards, while you are on vacation. This problem is more complicated than the first, but you eventually handle it by canceling the credit cards and duplicating the lost papers. If you can control the situation the stress produces, it is not harmful.

When individuals continually try to control an uncontrollable situation, they create problems for themselves. An executive who is fired, for instance, might continue to fight the situation for months, even to the point of taking the company to court. A driver stuck in traffic becomes impatient and rants and rages over the problems. Or a real estate broker may stew for days about a deal that fell through. All of these actions serve to create severe distress.

Richard S. Lazarus points out that an essential factor

in an individual's response to stress involves the person's appraisal of the situation and the manner in which the person copes with it. If complications of the situation don't outweigh the individual's ability to cope effectively, the effects of the stress are minimized. But when the coping is ineffective and the stress prolonged, the individual who still struggles against it may well make himself or herself sick.

No one knows if there is really more overall stress today than in the past, but many experts believe it has become more pervasive. "We live in a world of uncertainties," says Dr. Herbert Benson of Harvard, "everything from the nuclear threat, to corporation takeovers, to job insecurity, to worry over the economy and everything else."

TYPE A/TYPE B/TYPE C

How stress affects each individual, according to Meyer Friedman, M.D., depends on whether he or she is Type A or Type B. The most dramatic proof that stress is a direct contributing cause of heart disease was provided by Drs. Friedman and Ray H. Rosenman, who used behavior patterns to predict which subjects in a group of 3,500 would develop heart disease. After eight years of follow-up, they found that the hard-driving subjects, whom they labeled Type A, had more than twice as much heart disease as the more laid-back subjects they labeled Type B, who go through life at a sensible and relaxed pace.

Type A subjects had twice as much anginal pain, twice as many fatal heart attacks, five times as many recurring heart attacks, and twice as many heart events. Among subjects who died of other causes, the coronary arteries of the Type A subjects almost always showed far more disease than those of Type B subjects. Among the subjects considered the most relaxed and whose cholesterol level was under 225, not one had a heart attack.

I am very familiar with the work of Dr. Friedman and have spent many hours observing his cardiac rehabilitation and other programs. There is no question in my mind of the credibility of his research. And there is little doubt his programs have helped many to avoid coronary heart disease problems. Not all research supports the idea of a direct correlation between coronary heart disease and personality type, but can we afford to wait for the final verdict to change our manner of dealing with stress?

I identify with the plight of the Type A's. My wife is a definite Type B. When she discusses events of the day with me, I constantly interrupt, often finishing her sentences . . . which creates tension for both of us. I get irritated with cars ahead in line. I anguish at waiting to be seated in a restaurant. I am impatient with repetitious duties such as making out bank deposit slips. And in my business I hate filling out applications for clients.

According to Dr. Friedman, I am a typical Type A personality. This does not make me a unique individual, for this behavior afflicts at least 75 percent of American men and 40 to 50 percent of American women; Dr. Friedman's recent studies show that the ratio of Type A's to Type B's may be as high as 8 to 1 or even 10 to 1.

I am learning to be patient, but it is not easy. The behavior modification techniques taught me by Dr. Friedman have been a lifesaver and taught me to bring stress under control.

In terms of A's and B's, there are also overt A's. Overt A's have high drive, go at an accelerated pace, try to do too much in too little time, and are extremely competitive. But they nearly always tackle situations they can control. When they start out to solve a problem, they solve it. They, however, gradually give up on any situation in which they cannot win and further struggle will only result in frustration.

An insurance broker, for instance, might work frantically to write a policy. He does everything possible to make it work, he may get a bit frantic about it, but if he is an overt A, when he sees that it won't work, he walks away.

ARE YOU TYPE A OR TYPE B?

TYPE A BEHAVIOR CHARACTERISTICS

1. You feel a sense of time urgency—that there is not enough time to do all the things you wish to do.

2. You are impatient with the rate at which most events take place. You frequently hurry others' speech and interrupt others to finish their sentences.

3. You often think or try to do two or more things at the same time (called polyphasic thought or performance). This happens when you talk to someone about one thing but at the same time are thinking about another. When you do this, of course, you can't give the other person your undivided attention. A friend of mine brags that he can shave, read the newspaper, and get ready to go, all at the same time. You can often spot the Type A driver on the freeway using his electric razor or talking into her cellular phone.

4. You have difficulty just sitting and doing nothing. Many Type A's feel guilty when relaxing. Fortunately, I look forward to my quiet time each day, when I can work in the garden or walk, swim, or jog.

5. You have tense facial muscles—a facial expression of tension or anxiety.

6. You jiggle your knees or tap your fingers.

7. You frequently bring the conversation around to your interests.

8. You are unobservant of life's details and have little enjoyment of life.

9. You are always short of time and up against a deadline

and feel there's not enough time to do the things worth doing because of a preoccupation with the things worth having.

10. You believe that success is the ability to get things done faster than anyone else. You fear not being able to do things faster and faster.

11. You feel generalized hostility and aggression—excessive competitive drive.

- Explosively accentuating key words.

- Playing all games (even with children) to win.

- Clenching fists, pounding tables . . . forceful use of hands and fingers.

- Facial expression of aggression—clenching jaw, grinding of teeth.

- Irritation or rage when asked about past events that previously caused anger.

TYPE B BEHAVIOR CHARACTERISTICS

1. You have an absence of Type A habits or traits.

2. You do not feel time urgency and its accompanying impatience. In my 39 years of marriage, this is one area where my wife and I had a great deal of conflict. My Type B wife is always late. This creates stress for me, her Type A husband. During our dating period, she could never understand my being 20 to 30 minutes early.

3. You have no free-floating hostility; you don't need to display or discuss achievements or accomplishments.

4. You play for fun and relaxation, not for superiority.

5. You relax without guilt and work without agitation.

Behavior modification techniques can help the Type A make the transition to becoming a Type B. I work at it all the time. It is not easy, but it is worth the effort. No longer do I wear two watches; I often don't wear one. And I take time each day to relax. My productivity, instead of diminishing, has actually increased.

Adapted from M. Friedman and R. H. Rosenman, *Treating Type A Behavior and Your Heart* (New York: Alfred A. Knopf, 1984).

A number of people have developed incredible coping abilities, self-control, and personal strength. The results of this are not only increased mental and emotional strength and vigor, but also an enhanced ability to relax, stay calm, and be positive even under pressure.

When confronted with a stressful situation, the first reaction of the members of this group is one of calm reason and determination rather than resentment. These people recognize they can't afford to feel personally threatened by or even too concerned about the problem. Instead they take a lighthearted attitude, which seems to insulate them from the negative effects of stress.

One of the most notable examples of this quality is former president Ronald Reagan. Even with the stresses of running the country, Reagan always displayed the ability to let stress "roll off his back" while retaining a jovial attitude. In contrast, the stress of the presidency aged Jimmy Carter considerably during his four years in office, and Richard Nixon attributes the dangerous blood clots he experienced to the stress of Watergate.

The type A personality is pretty well established as aggressive and impatient, and the Type B personality as one who takes things more in stride and seems to enjoy life more without overexertion.

Now medical researchers are talking about the Type C personality (the C stands for cancer). Lydia Temoshok, a psychologist at the University of California, San Francisco, says that Type C's are completely opposite to the hard-driving, get-out-of-my-way Type A's. These patients afflicted with melanoma were supercooperative, nice to a fault, and without a visible trace of hostility. Their feelings are so far beneath the surface that they have lost awareness of how they really do feel. The energy required to prevent feelings from bubbling to the surface, Temoshok says, may weaken the system and open the door to cancer. When asked about the difficulty of coping, these individuals passed off the idea as being related to other people.

Cancer patients who talked about past emotional experience, discussed their feelings openly, and actively sought to overcome their disease had a far greater survival rate than patients with a stoic attitude.

Many researchers also now believe that cancer, arthritis, ulcerated colitis, asthma, migraine headaches, and numerous psychosomatic disorders are associated with very distinct personality types and specific clusters of personality traits.

STRESS AND HEART ATTACKS

Dr. Friedman's researchers have found that Type A victims have more of the so-called "struggle" hormone, norepinephrine, circulating in their bloodstream than non–Type A's. Norepinephrine is now regarded by researchers throughout the world as playing an even greater role than dietary cholesterol in the development of coronary heart disease. According to Walter Schafer, who heads a stress center at the Enloe Memorial Hospital in Chico, California, norepinephrine contributes to a higher heart rate, hypertension, and insulin-induced damage to coronary walls, as well as increasing cholesterol flow in the blood.

Reporting on his studies with animals, Baylor University physiologist Dr. James E. Skinner stated, "Having a blood clot in a coronary artery does not cause you to die. A psychological stress factor needs to be present." Dr. Skinner's laboratory blocked the coronary arteries of two groups of pigs, the animal whose cardiovascular system is most like that of humans. One group was subjected to stress, the other was not. The animals under stress experienced a high death rate, while none of the other animals died, even though the major blood supply to their hearts was blocked. The psychological factor of stress was necessary for the blockage of the coronary artery to produce ventricular fibrillation, the death-causing rhythmical disorder of heart attacks.

Ventricular fibrillation is a kind of wild fluttering of the heart muscle in place of the regular contractions that normally enable it to pump blood to the brain and other parts of the body. Reported Skinner, "It may be that brain activity alone is sufficient to cause the initiation of ventricular fibrillation without coronary blockage."

THE HOSTILITY FACTOR

Everyone is burdened with some form of hidden anger and resentment that in turn expresses itself negatively in his or her life. Hidden anger tends to seep into our daily experience without our knowledge.

Once the anger is lodged in the subconscious, it seems to take over. Studies by Redford B. Williams, Jr., of the Duke University Medical Center in Durham, North Carolina, suggest that high scores on a psychological test designed to measure hostility are associated with high risk of heart disease from all causes. These studies show that it is not the hard-driving workaholic who is at risk, but the hard-driving workaholic who is also angry, hostile, and distrustful.

His research also found that a study group of doctors with high scores on a hostility test given during medical school were more likely to die during the 25-year follow-up period than were their more relaxed peers. Only 2 percent of physicians with low or average hostility scores died, while 14 percent of physicians with above average hostility died during the same period.

In a related study, researchers followed a group of 118 lawyers who were given the Minnesota Multiphasic Personality Inventory test. Twenty years later those with the higher hostility scores died at a rate 412 times higher than those with low scores.

Williams believes hostility is the critical component of the Type A personality and a potent predictor of heart trouble. Hostile people are more likely to meet daily challenges with large increases in blood pressure. The Type A might get extremely angry if a customer ahead of him in the supermarket express line has 15 items in his basket instead of the permitted 10 and might even go so far as to complain about it out loud to the checkout clerk or manager. Such situations that just annoy the average person, in the hostile Type A person may produce not only sharp increases in blood pressure but also a surge of adrenaline that is equivalent to the amount produced during heavy exercise. The extra adrenaline, however, is not burned up but instead releases fatty acids that clog arteries.

Driving is especially hazardous to the health of the Type A driver. You can observe him as he speeds down the highway, tooting his horn at slower drivers, tailgating, and rolling through stop signs.

"A lot of people," said Dr. Malcolm Carruthers, "are driving themselves to death." Dr. Carruthers, a research pathologist, and Dr. Peter Toggert, a cardiologist, measured the heart rates of two groups of London commuters, one with a history of heart trouble and one supposedly fit. The heart of a fit man at rest beats about 70 times a minute. After extreme prolonged exercise, the heart rate may rise as high as 210. The two doctors found that by the time the drivers had reached work the hearts of the fit men had sped up to 100–155, while those of the unfit men had reached 180—the same level recorded for racing drivers after a Grand Prix. In both groups, the body produced extra adrenalin as it does during strong exercise. I often think of this when I feel tension mount while I am stuck in traffic. I know the healthy thing to do would be to get out and jog around my car to burn up the fatty acids, but I doubt if this act would be tolerated.

WORK-RELATED STRESS

The workplace is filled with stress-related mental health problems. The majority of medical directors of major companies report that this type of health problem is either very pervasive or fairly pervasive at their own company. In the workplace, stress exacts both a psychological and an economic toll.

According to a Gallup survey, each year 29 percent of the corporate work force suffers from anxiety disorders or a stress-related illness. Each stressed-out employee loses an average of 16 days of work each year because of mental health problems.

A Gallup Poll of 210 personnel and medical directors of America's corporations found that stress-related depression may affect up to 24 percent of the work force.

It is predicted that the number of stress-related workers' compensation claims will continue to grow at current rates during the 1990s. Stress-related mental disorders are now being called the country's fastest-growing occupational disease. And the cost of occupational disability related to anxiety, depression, and stress will be about $8,000 per case.

Stress/Distress in the Workplace

The stress/distress concept has proved to be an extremely accurate predictor of destructive stress in the workplace. For instance, studies based on a million male and female Swedish workers found that heart disease is more prevalent in workers whose jobs combine heavy demands with little ability to influence how their tasks are done. Dr. Robert Karasek, Ph.D., associate professor of industrial and systems engineering at the University of Southern California, who conducted the studies with colleagues in Sweden and at Columbia University, found in another study of 15,000 male workers that individuals with little control over their jobs are four times as likely to suffer heart attacks as those with a high degree of job control. The average rate of heart attacks among American working men is currently 2 percent. But Dr. Karasek discovered that male American workers with high job control and low psychological demands had half that rate and men with low job control and high psychological demands had twice that rate of heart attacks. "The health risk of low job control," says Dr. Karasek, "is

---

THE CORONARY CLUB

People who live with a lot of stress are at higher risk for cardiovascular incidence. The set of questions below can help you determine if you are eligible for membership in this exclusive club.

1. Do you tend to go to the office on Saturdays, evenings, and holidays?

2. Do you take your briefcase home at night and review your troubles and worries?

3. Do you show up early in the morning after a late-night meeting to impress the office staff?

4. Are meals often hurried and tense?

5. Do you often do business at lunch?

6. Do you consider fishing, hunting, golf, and other leisure activities a waste of time?

7. Do you keep in touch with the office during vacation?

8. Do you have difficulty delegating authority?

9. When traveling, is your motto "Work all day and drive all night"?

10. Do you spend inordinate amounts of time on outside activities, join committees, and accept invitations to most banquets?

11. In addition to your regular work, do you sit up half the night writing reports?

Source: "The Coronary Club," *Life Association News,* December 1986, p. 17.

roughly of the same magnitude as the risk from smoking or high serum cholesterol."

The Responsibility of Work

Research now shows that the more you resent the responsibility of work, the more oversensitive you become to it as a pressure. This is the pressure we often feel as workplace distress. Reacting to this stress generates more resentment, which creates even greater stress. The job can then start to become overwhelming as the normal responsibilities and problems of work become magnified in your mind. The result of this cycle can be greater inefficiency on the job, depression, job burnout, a nervous breakdown, and sometimes a heart attack.

This realization is not new. Dr. Henry I. Russek, while cardiovascular consultant to the United States Public Health Service Hospital at Staten Island, concluded that job-related emotional stress might be a far more significant factor in heart disease than heredity, dietary fat, tobacco, obesity, or physical activity, although he did not minimize the importance of these other factors.

The Inability to Express Yourself

People who can't express themselves to authority figures are supersensitive to all pressures and extremely resentful! They become very angry and are unable to cope with stress. A most dangerous situation, especially if other factors such as smoking, obesity, high blood pressure, and physical inactivity are present.

People Who Stress Others

Other people have an unhealthy drive to succeed. They make success the most important thing in their lives to the emotional detriment of themselves and their families. Sometimes they seem well adjusted and outgoing. Members of this group, however, have large unhealthy egos. They draw their total identity and sense of self-worth from who they know, how much money they earn, and what other people say about them. They are preoccupied with material things and acceptance and admiration from others. As children they most likely wanted to be the first one on the block with a new bicycle. They gathered toys, not only to play with but to show off to others. Now they acquire office buildings, shopping centers, stocks, bonds, and other evidence of wealth. The recognition they receive from this compensates for deep feelings of emptiness and inadequacy.

These people create considerable stress for people around them as they have a compulsion to dominate, psychologically and monetarily. They are a danger to the health of others as well as themselves.

Stress of Success

Business can be a caldron of pressure that can make or break a person's ability to deal with stress. In the many years I've been in the sales field, I've been surprised by the number of young people who fail even though they're intelligent and alert and have good looks and a pleasant personality. In talking to them and observing their behavior, I've come to the conclusion that it is their inability to handle stress that causes their downfall in fields in which they should exel.

Even the most well-adjusted person who has achieved success in life as a manager or the owner of a business is constantly assaulted with a whole array of problems and stresses that most people don't have to deal with. A common misconception related to stress, however, is that it is mainly the executives who suffer stress-related health problems. We usually visualize a high-powered sales executive as pacing up and down in front of his or her desk, talking into two phones at once while dictating to a secretary.

A study by Metropolitan Life Insurance Company, however, concluded that top executives of both leading corporations and smaller businesses actually have a longer life expectancy than other American men. In one study top executives in 50 leading companies had a 37 percent lower mortality rate than other employees in those same companies.

A 1963 study of 86,000 Du Pont employees verifies this. Top executives had the lowest ratio of heart attacks, blue-collar workers the highest. Dr. Lawrence E. Hinkle, head of the Division of Human Ecology, Cornell University Medical College, New York, studying 270,000 employees of the Bell Telephone Company, found that the number of heart attacks there had relatively little to do with how hard a person worked or with the tensions and responsibilities of his or her position.

The reason for this, these studies conclude, is that most top executives are under stress, not distress. While the executives face considerable pressures each day, they for the most part solve these problems and go on to handle others. The bottom line is that while they are under pressure, they also retain some control over these pressures, a fact, again, researchers say makes all the difference in the world.

These and other studies suggest the conclusion that stress itself has little if any connection with heart disease. University of Michigan neurophysiologist Dr. Ralph W. Gerard declared, "Activity of the nervous system improves its capacity for activity just as exercising a muscle makes it stronger."

Distress, contends Dr. Robert Elliot, professor of medicine and director of the Cardiovascular Center at the University of Nebraska Medical Center, "can be a killer unless we learn to recognize it and effectively cope with it." What can kill you, he tells his patients, is hostility, impatience, and competitiveness, which increase the blood vessels' peripheral resistance to the heartbeat, "acting just like a clamp being forced down on a garden hose. The heart must under these conditions pump against dramatically increased pressure, and there's a limit to what it can do."

Stressed-Out Occupations

A number of occupations seem to create additional stress-related health problems for individuals within that profession. Dr. Elliot investigated stress at Cape Kennedy and discovered that aerospace workers there, some as young as 29, sometimes died of stress-induced heart attacks when they learned their jobs were being phased out. The engineers and technicians there, average age 31, also had almost a 50 percent higher rate of sudden death than matched controls. This he associated with the demanding schedules and the possibility of being laid off after the mission was accomplished. The study also found that these workers had a high rate of alcohol abuse and divorce. Autopsies showed that some of these young professionals' heart muscles had been ruptured in seconds by a stress-induced outpouring of catecholamine.

Other occupations, he discovered, such as air traffic controllers, are at risk. These controllers have five to six times more hypertension than a comparison group of aviation workers.

Dr. Elliot maintains that this distress is caused by a number of risk factors. But very specific events can increase the risk. For instance, he reports that of the 1,200 sudden cardiac deaths a week in the United States, almost half, 43 percent, occur on a Monday. Similarly, Friedman and Rosenman found that accountants have abnormally high blood cholesterol counts during abnormally stressful periods. In January, when they close out their clients' books, and in March and early April, when they are preparing tax returns, they are especially prone to heart atacks.

According to Dr. Elliot's study, today's women are more stressed than men. Not only has women's liberation brought more women into new arenas and new stresses, but many are still expected to remain feminine, motherly, loving, and nonthreatening to men. And it's not only in the workplace that stress takes its toll on women. Researchers at the 1985 American Psychological Association's meeting reported that housewives with driven personalities feel the same stress, fear, and dissatisfaction associated with career men and women with Type A personalities.

At the age of 44, Dr. Elliot had a heart attack while lecturing on how to prevent heart attacks. He was a nonsmoker, was not overweight, did not have high blood pressure, and had parents who lived to a ripe old age. He attributes his attack to a life that "had been a blur of overachievement to gain recognition." He now recommends to everyone to cope with modern pressures by relaxation, and suggests, "Rule number one is don't sweat the small stuff. Rule number two is, it's all small stuff. And if you can't fight and you can't flee, flow."

Company Involvement

Currently the estimated cost of stress to companies ranges from $12,550 per employee to as much as $1 million for top executives who die of premature heart disease. As a result a number of companies have begun to build on-premise exercise facilities and to sponsor meditation classes and biofeedback programs.

Equitable Life Assurance Society claims to have saved $5,152 in medical costs for every dollar invested. New York Telephone instituted a program with periodic health exams for all employees and meditation lessons for those with stress-related symptoms. This has helped cut the corporate hypertension rate from 18 percent— about average for U.S. firms—to half that amount. One pioneering firm based in Great Neck, New York, with 300 employees, is even building an executive retreat in Vero Beach, Florida, expressly for use as a stress-reduction center.

HOW VULNERABLE ARE YOU TO STRESS?

This test was developed by psychologists Lyle H. Miller and Alma Dell Smith at Boston University Medical Center. Score each item from 1 (almost always) to 5 (never), according to how much of the time each statement applies to you.

____ 1. I eat at least one hot, balanced meal a day.

____ 2. I get seven to eight hours sleep at least four nights a week.

____ 3. I give and receive affection regularly.

____ 4. I have at least one relative within 50 miles on whom I can rely.

____ 5. I exercise to the point of perspiration at least twice a week.

____ 6. I smoke less than half a pack of cigarettes a day.

____ 7. I take fewer than five alcoholic drinks a week.

____ 8. I am the appropriate weight for my height.

____ 9. I have an income adequate to meet basic expenses.

____ 10. I get strength from my religious beliefs.

____ 11. I regularly attend club or social activities.

____ 12. I have a network of friends and acquaintances.

____ 13. I have one or more friends to confide in about personal matters.

____ 14. I am in good health (including eyesight, hearing, teeth).

____ 15. I am able to speak openly about my feelings when angry or worried.

____ 16. I have regular conversations with the people I live with about domestic problems, e.g., chores, money, and daily living issues.

____ 17. I do something for fun at least once a week.

____ 18. I am able to organize my time effectively.

____ 19. I drink fewer than three cups of coffee (or tea or cola drinks) a day.

____ 20. I take quiet time for myself during the day.

____ TOTAL

To get your score, add up the figures and subtract 20. Any number over 30 indicates a vulnerability to stress. You are seriously vulnerable if your score is between 50 and 75, and extremely vulnerable if it is over 75.

LETTING GO OF STRESS

Strong negative emotions are responsible for self-destructive behavioral patterns. Jumping to conclusions, condemning others, being cruel to or hating those who are cruel to you—these are the things that exact a high price in terms of physical and mental well-being. But they are also responses you can actually control and eliminate.

Unless people recognize and deal with these internal emotional mechanisms, they will always blame people, places, and things for distress. However, deadlines, pressure from bosses, money problems, and angry spouses are not the causes of distress. Rather it is how you as an individual react to these things that causes physical problems.

Often it is not possible to change your job, your environment, or your current situation as a means of eliminating stress. And even if you do, the same stresses may crop up again in other situations. Fortunately, research has shown that it is only necessary to change yourself and the way you relate to stress to really make a difference. Harry Truman used to say, "If you can't stand the heat, get out of the kitchen." During the last days of World War II, President Truman was asked how he managed to bear up so calmly under the stresses of the presidency. "I have a foxhole in my mind," he replied, explaining that just as a soldier retreats into his foxhole for protection and respite, he periodically retreated into his mental "foxhole" where he allowed nothing to bother him. In doing so, he was following the wisdom of Marcus Aurelius, who wrote, "Nowhere either with more quiet or more freedom from trouble does a man retire more than into his own soul."

What can you do to get rid of the anger, hatred, rage, frustration, envy, apathy, and cynicism that create the problem hostility? The key to this seems to be forgiveness of both yourself and those who consciously or unconsciously are cruel or unreasonable or just get in your way.

Patience is the character strength that prevents others from upsetting you and getting under your skin. And when others try to get to you, true patience deflects their attempts. Through patience and forgiveness and the strength of compassion, you can not only resolve your distress problems, but also help those around you who are caught in the powerful grip of their own negative emotions.

If stress is a problem for you, you can often let go of stress and minimize its harmful consequences by following a few simple guidelines:

1. Watch for signs of stress: nervousness, increased muscle tension, migraine headaches, ulcers, high blood pressure, chest pains, severe nervousness, depression, or extreme mental confusion.

2. Consciously minimize the source of your concern. Engage in some activity that holds your attention. Even watching television can work.

3. Practice defocused concentration 5 to 30 minutes a day. With relaxing music or taped sounds of the ocean in the background, focus your attention simultaneously on two or more points of the body, the right hand and the center of the forehead, or both hands and the forehead. Try to resist the natural tendency for your mind to wander. When this exercise is done correctly it helps clear the mind, leading to relaxation of the muscles, deeper and slower breathing, and, after about 5 to 15 minutes, a very pleasant sensation of lightness and relaxation. See Figure 6-4 for a more detailed description.

4. Remove or reduce external sources of stress. Hopelessness is a condition wherein people honestly believe that nothing can be done about their situation or rela-

RELAXATION EXERCISE

This stress-reducing exercise is recognized, used, and endorsed by many practicing psychologists and psychiatrists for individuals who want to reduce anxiety.

1. Sit in a comfortable chair and relax. Drop both hands into your lap or at your sides.

2. Consciously think about your right hand. Just be aware that it is there.

3. Anytime you direct your attention to any part of your body, you will get a reaction. As you remain aware of your hand, it will begin to tingle and then feel warm. Notice any thought that begins to distract you. If a thought draws your attention away from your hand, simply redirect your attention to your hand. Become aware of it so that you feel it glow warmly.

4. Now shift your attention from one finger to another. Be aware of the thumb, then shift the feeling to your first finger, then the second, the third, and the little finger. Begin again. You should soon feel energy flowing down your arm, into your hand, and then through the body.

5. Continue being aware of your hand/body glowing warmly. If a thought pulls you into a daydream or worry, pull back and observe the feeling of your hand and body.

6. Now see if you can put a distance between you and objects close to you. Detach yourself. Just observe any distractions or memories, and keep your thoughts on the warmth of your body.

---

tionship. By patiently and unemotionally observing the actions of those who are exerting pressure on you, you will gradually see what you must do to improve the situation.

5. Exercise. Even a minimal amount of regular exercise can improve your health, longevity, and resistance to stress. A sedentary person who begins an exercise

program that he or she enjoys, and continues it week after week, will most likely obtain dramatic improvements in his or her stress-fitness. There is no definite prescription for exercise—find the exercise you enjoy and that suits your lifestyle, whether it be walking, bicycling, dancing, jogging, or whatever. Generally the experts recommend exercising three times a week.

I often rely on exercise to help me handle stress. I realized this when a life insurance company I had helped found started to falter. In less than a month I experienced a paper loss of almost half a million dollars. I found myself constantly reassuring stockholders that the company was solid, its production increasing (no, I did not unload my shares). After a long run and a cold shower, I could cope. I, like many others, have found exercise a great tranquilizer in times of stress. See Chapter 2 for a complete exercise program.

6. **Eat right.** The link between diet and mental and emotional well-being has been established through research and validated through personal experience. Proper nutrition, an important component of an overall stress-reduction plan, promotes a more youthful feeling and appearance, while improper eating habits create obesity, poor complexion, and loss of energy— adding an unnecessary stress to the entire system.

7. **Get a pet.** Erika Friedman, Ph.D., associate professor, Brooklyn College, finds that pets have a tranquilizing effect that markedly lowers the heart rates of Type A participants in her research. Regular contact with pets, she reports, can provide direct health benefits by reducing stress. Pets provide companionship and love and help calm individuals down.

8. **Laugh.** Laughter also helps reduce stress. Medical

research now suggests that it gives a workout to bodily organs and triggers the secretion of endorphins in the brain, which fosters a sense of relaxation and well-being and dulls the perception of pain. Dr. William Fry, a psychiatrist affiliated with Stanford University and a student of laughter for three decades, says laughing 100 times a day is equivalent to about 10 minutes of rowing. As Dr. Marvin Eitterring of the New Jersey School of Osteopathic Medicine puts it, the thorax, heart, lungs, diaphragm, abdomen, and even the liver are given a massage during a hearty laugh. I often thought that laughter had something to do with the longevity of famous comedians such as Eddie Cantor, Jack Benny, Myron Cohen, George Jessel, George Burns, and Bob Hope. I am sure that President Reagan's sense of humor has helped to sustain him through many complicated events.

9. Build a network of friends. The physical and psychological benefits of support from friends and family can be dramatic. Studies conducted over a nine-year period in Alameda County, California, for example, have indicated that people who have extensive networks of social support may live longer than those who do not. Social support can reduce stress symptoms following the loss of a loved one, help speed recovery from surgery and heart attacks, and alleviate the symptoms of asthma and other disorders. Good friends are essential for good health. While surveying unemployed workers in the Detroit area, University of Michigan Researcher Louis Ferman found one hard-luck victim who had been successively laid off by the Studebaker Corp. in 1962 when it was about to fold, a truck manufacturer that went under in the 1970s, and more recently during cutbacks at a Chrysler plant. By all accounts, "he should

have been a basket case," says Ferman, "yet he was one of the best-adjusted fellows I've run into." Asked his secret, the man replied, "I've got a loving wife and go to church every Sunday."

Stress, of course, is never listed as the official cause of a fatal heart attack, yet its danger is undisputed. Not only traffic but many other "acts of daily living" create tremendous amounts of distress. Many physicians today estimate mental stress has either caused or aggravated the symptoms of 50 to 90 percent of all inpatients. This includes patients with ulcers, cancer, stroke, heart disease, migraine headaches, hypertension, and many other problems. With care, however, stress can be brought under control and made to work for, not against, you.

7
Recovering from a Heart Attack

Thanks to major breakthroughs in the area of heart disease, many people who already have had a heart attack or stroke and were fortunate enough to survive can look forward to a long and healthy life. One day they may even look back at the illness as a blessing in disguise. Mother Nature's warning can cause you to sit up and notice that you were not taking good care of your circulatory system, not eating properly, not exercising or relaxing enough, not listening to that cigarette cough.

"The name of the game in heart attacks," says cardiologist James Schoendezer, former president of the American Heart Association and professor of preventive medicine at Chicago's Rush–Presbyterian–St. Luke's Medical Center, "is learning how to avoid the next one." Actually, when you think of it, the first heart attack, when you survive it, is one of the body's chief warning devices that tells you to shape up, now, or drop dead!

Although your body is a wondrous creation, if you don't take care of it, you should expect something to give. If you've heard Mother Nature's warning, you'd better change your ways. Remember, if you want to play the game, you have to follow the rules. For those who do, the outlook is surprisingly bright.

Not too long ago, doctors would tell people who'd had heart attacks that they'd have to take it easy for the rest of their days. "Don't run if you can walk; if you have to walk, count to 10 between steps; don't walk if you can sit down; don't sit down if you can lie down." As late as 1956 a medical textbook recommended that a heart patient be restricted to walking short distances and playing croquet.

Sadly, I recall how my father was told to curtail all physical activity after his first heart attack. This advice most likely contributed to his demise one year later.

Studies have shown that this approach is a dangerous one, and many cardiologists feel that recovery really is complete when the patient gives up living in fear and resumes his normal life. In one sanitarium, patients were divided into two groups—the sitters, who convalesced on the veranda, and the walkers, who hiked over nearby hills. At the end of one year, half the sitters were dead, while most of the walkers were alive and well.

Dr. Herman Hellerstein of the Case Western Reserve School of Medicine in Cleveland has shown that physical exercise may be of real benefit to heart patients. When 656 middle-aged men were put on an active conditioning program involving weight control, diet therapy, cessation of smoking, and regular exercise, a subgroup of 100 men with coronary heart disease was able to perform muscular effort with fewer heartbeats, lower blood pressure, and greater aerobic capacity than before training. Studies in the 1970s showed that the care of heart attack patients in the period emphasized less dependence on bed rest and an increase in physical activity. Progress in cardiac rehabilitation, according to Dr. Nanette Wenger of the Emory University School of Medicine in Atlanta, Georgia, demands that the patient after a heart attack or coronary bypass surgery be "integrated into a comprehensive program of acute and ambulatory cardiac care." That's something for the sitters who have sustained a heart attack to think about.

Although the reasons heart patients benefit from physical exercise aren't fully understood, there is agreement that these patients need no longer spend their lives feeling like invalids or social has-beens. If you say to your body, "I've had it, I no longer can get around well, feel good, perform sexually, and enjoy life," that's exactly what will happen. But if you say, "Thanks for the warning. This will be a new beginning. With this rude awakening, I'm going to become a new person," then you'll become happier and healthier.

Among the people who feel their heart attack was a fortunate thing is a retired Sacramento printer who thought he had less than a year to live. Since he didn't have a suit to be buried in, he went out and bought one for a hundred dollars. Then, on a whim, he also purchased a bicycle. The bicycle became a very important part of his life. Riding between 20 and 40 miles a day since his heart attack, he has cycled more than 70,000 miles, shed 40 pounds, and worn out the suit he was supposed to be buried in. As his wife of 45 years declared, "If it hadn't been for that bike, he'd be out there in his grave. It's made him feel useful rather than just sitting around waiting to die."

In contrast, a client of mine who had a heart attack at the age of 48 had to give up his job and go on a full disability pension because of his health. Although his doctor warned him to stop smoking, watch his weight, and get on a mild exercise program, sadly he did just the opposite. He continued smoking, gained weight, and, as his widow said, did nothing but lie around and feel sorry for himself. Two years later he had a fatal heart attack, leaving his wife to raise their children alone.

Eula Weaver is a wonderful example of a person who has listened to her physician and learned to live with a coronary problem. At the age of 88, she had 10 years earlier had a stroke that left her partially paralyzed, and she was suffering from hypertension, angina, and arthritis. But instead of giving up, she started on an exercise program that had dramatic results. As she tells it, "My doctor gave me two choices: either to spend the rest of my life as an invalid being fed and clothed, or to begin walking again, no matter how painful it would be." Her decision came quickly: "I vowed then and there that I'd try everything in the world that would help get me back to normal."

She started to walk a little each day, gradually increasing the distance to at least six miles. She also went on a strict diet of green vegetables, fresh raw fruit, less than three ounces of meat a day, and no salt, sugar, coffee, tea, or alcohol. Soon she was so physically fit she began jogging two miles a day. In 1975, she entered the National Senior Olympics. She is the sole competitor over 80 years of age in the 1,500-meter run for women and has won the championship each year. Now that she is nearing 90, her daily two-mile jog has been reduced to one mile. If it rains, she rides the stationary bicycle in her living room and pedals 10 miles or so. She also visits a local gym three times a week.

Another good example of a heart patient following his doctor's advice is a Cleveland businessman who joined a YMCA. His story is typical. He had been a high school star athlete and later a weight lifter. As he became involved in business, he neglected to exercise and eventually had a king-sized heart attack. After a series of tests, he was advised to run a little, swim a little, and work up gradually. Although he was very reluctant to accept this advice, he knew others had followed it with success.

With great care and patience, the Y staff led him progressively through more difficult grades of jogging, swimming, and calisthenics. In four months, his pulse had dropped from 98 to 58. His blood pressure dropped too. On his 63rd birthday he ran 10 miles in an hour and 17 minutes, and a year later he clipped six minutes off his record. His run was covered by local TV, radio, and press reporters. What a shame that this inspiring story didn't have national coverage so that it could encourage other heart patients.

Similar programs exist all over the country. The formula is a supervised program that is based on increasing the patients' activities until they reach an optimum level. Physiologist Dr. Thomas Cureton of the University of Illinois School of Physical Fitness told me they have had some patients in their program who were in such bad shape that they started by doing nothing more than walking in chest-deep water from one side of the pool to the other. They gradually worked up to a program that included 40 minutes of limbering-up calisthenics, one mile of jogging, and a mile or more of swimming every day. I have interviewed many cardiac patients in various rehabilitation programs and even jogged alongside them. There is no doubt in my mind of the tremendous progress they are making.

More objective testimony is presented by the x-rays and cardiograms documenting the changes in these rejuvenated hearts. One study compared these heart patients with a group of businessmen going to the YMCA on a casual basis to play volleyball or basketball, swim, or jog around the track. In cardiorespiratory tests, the cardiac patients on a consistent supervised program did better than the businessmen.

These results are not surprising to Dr. Terence Kavanagh, director of the Toronto Rehabilitation Centre. In a 1975 study of 40 patients on a combined exercise and diet program, 6 showed for the first time what is called "plaque reversal." This evidence suggests that if such a program is started before the fatty deposits of atherosclerosis harden, the condition may be reversible.

A few of the post–heart attack patients in Dr. Kavanagh's distance jogging program eventually run marathon distances. He permits prospective joggers to enter his program only after they have taken a stress test to determine their readiness for physical activity. Depending on the results of the test, he will prescribe walking, jogging, or running to recondition these patients to normal lives.

Developed as an experiment in community postcoronary rehabilitation, the program has enrolled close to 1,000 patients, and 17 have run in over 50 cross-country races, including the Boston and Hawaii marathons. After several years of reconditioning, one of his patients finished the 26-mile, 385-yard Boston Marathon in three hours and 17 minutes—nine minutes better than the doctor.

Dr. Kavanagh says that although he never could guarantee anyone immunity against heart attack, his program is very successful in forestalling repeat attack. The results can be seen most dramatically in the few men who have progressed through the various stages of jogging and graduated into the marathon division. "They aren't the men who, at first glance, you would think would graduate to this level," he says. One 47-year-old with severe heart disease and angina attacks completed the Hawaii Marathon in five hours and 45 minutes.

Dr. Kavanagh points out that there have been 12 deaths from heart attacks in the Toronto jogging programs, none of them at the marathon level and most among smokers and early in the program's history. He stresses that it is essential before a patient goes out onto the track that he undergo, in addition to a thorough physical, a thorough examination by a clinical psychologist. His studies have indicated that a third of the patients suffer from severe depression without overt symptoms and need a good deal of encouragement to run fast enough to allay their fears.

He also is concerned about those in the nondepressed group who are ambitious, driving, competitive, overcommitted, and full of concealed hostility. These people tend to want to prove immediately that their heart attack hasn't slowed them down and will aim for an eight-minute mile if you expect them to run it in nine. They either follow Dr. Kavanagh's instructions or are dropped from the program. Currently Dr. Kavanagh's work is receiving considerable recognition. The Japanese are most interested in applying his cardiac rehabilitation services to those already affected by coronary artery disease.

Cardiologist Dr. Jack H. Scall, Jr., started Honolulu's Central YMCA Cardiac Rehabilitation Program in 1973, a program I am personally familiar with. A past president of the Honolulu Marathon Association, Scall had 50 heart patients in training for a marathon run. His basic program calls for an hour's running three times a week, which, he said, "has about the same effect on the cardiovascular system as six hours of singles tennis. The heart shows no deterioration in a marathon run, and it is extremely safe if it is run in an appropriate setting."

If this makes you want to work up to one of these long-distance events to prevent a heart attack or a repeat attack, listen carefully to the lifesaving advice of a pioneer in this kind of program: Since every individual is different, so his or her exercise needs are different. Before any middle-aged, out-of-condition person decides to exercise, that person should consult his or her family doctor. The doctor should review the patient's medical history, give him or her a thorough physical examination, and make needed laboratory tests. If free of organic disease, the patient may be permitted to start an individualized program of the types available in many YMCAs. But he or she should start slowly and exercise regularly, increasing the work load gradually. Such a program is useful for anyone who is overweight or who has a family history of vascular disease. But get your doctor's advice first.

I would add to this that it helps to consult a cardiologist who is aware of and receptive to the new cardiac rehabilitation programs. Being involved at the voluntary level with such programs, I've had the opportunity to observe and evaluate several that were offered privately and others offered as a service in hospitals and other health agencies. I've been very much impressed by the leadership involved and by the enthusiasm of the participants. A recent study of aerobic exercise indicates the benefits that heart patients and others can derive from these programs.

As to the value of physical activity programs following a heart attack, the final verdict may not be in yet, but there are many strong, long-term supporters of this concept, such as Dr. William Haskell, co-director, Stanford Cardiac Rehabilitation Program, who states, "Selected patients, after acute myocardial infarction, have benefited from appropriate increases in physical activity. They have had fewer complications associated with bed rest, made a more successful psychological adjustment to their disease, shown improved cardiovascular function and physical working capacity, returned to gainful employment earlier and more frequently, and had fewer and less severe reinfarctions."

A more recent study by G. T. O'Connor and associates found that exercise training increases the likelihood of survival for at least three years after a heart attack and that if these programs were available nationwide they might well save approximately 13,000 lives annually. The study further concludes it is reasonable to assume that middle-aged men in exercise-based rehabilitation programs after myocardial infarction can anticipate enhanced survival as a result of this exercise training.

According to a recent committee editorial report, the cost is minimal when compared with the billions of dollars spent on palliation of vascular complications of atherosclerosis. Limiting the growth of cardiac rehabilitation programs can only increase the burden of atherosclerotic disease and the costs of high-tech treatments. But just as we have discovered in the earlier chapters, exercise programs will not do it alone. In fact, as valuable as physical activity is to the recovery of the heart, several reports stress the importance of adding other treatments. This is a good reason for you, if you have had a heart attack, to contact local hospitals, the YMCA, and other sources to find a good nearby cardiac rehabilitation program. Make certain that, in addition to exercise, they offer nutritional counseling and, most important, counseling to modify Type A behavior.

The program developed by Diane Ulmer and Dr. Meyer Friedman has produced dramatic reduction in the rate of cardiac recurrence. No drug, food, or exercise program ever devised, not even coronary bypass surgery, has matched the protection against recurrent heart attacks that this behavioral counseling program has achieved.

While serving as chairman of a cardiac rehabilitation committee, I spent several days at the Mt. Zion Hospital and Medical Center in San Francisco observing their program and was most favorably impressed by the spectacular results. To make a coronary comeback, it is just what the doctor ordered. The findings of a 44-year study of over 1,000 men and women (all of whom survived at least one heart attack) are discussed in Friedman and Ulmer's book *Treating Type A Behavior and Your Heart* (New York: Alfred A. Knopf, 1984). Many victims have a tough time coping with a heart attack. Fortunately the stigma that once existed is fading. For the close to a million people a year who survive, the road to recovery may be tough, but it is not impossible.

The shift from hospital to home and from home to the workplace is also challenging and traumatic. Usually the patients are chronically tired and easily fatigued. They normally feel depressed and tend to assume the worst. The cardiac rehabilitation programs certainly help with that transition. They are a must, for if you continue the same lifestyle that caused the first heart attack, a second one may very well occur.

SEX AND A HEART ATTACK

Most patients are fearful of sexual activity after a heart attack. But contrary to common belief, sexual activity is the norm and not dangerous. As expected after a heart attack, the patient may very well lose interest in sex for a while and also be reluctant to express his or her fears.

Sometimes the partners are reluctant to make love because they fear a heart attack during sex. Surprisingly, the fear of having intercourse can be as much of a risk factor for a coronary artery attack as sex itself.

Yet in the early 1970s, researchers in Cleveland were able to document that sex with someone you have had a long and stable relationship with is entirely safe. The energy expended while having sex is simply equivalent to the energy it takes to climb one flight of stairs. In another study, conducted by the Japanese, the investigators obtained and analyzed the autopsy records of 5,000 people who had died suddenly. Of this group, 34 had died during intercourse; of the 34, 30 were with someone other than their spouse, and the partner was on average 18 years younger. Moreover, all had blood alcohol levels close to or within the range of intoxication. The results are not conclusive but suggest that extramarital affairs, especially those involving a younger partner, produce more and potentially lethal stress.

GOING BACK TO WORK

Cardiac programs have helped show industry leaders that a heart attack need not mean that a person's active days are over. Union Carbide discovered during medical examinations that some employees had evidence of earlier heart disease that they either hadn't recognized or had failed to report to the company when they were hired. "We were greatly impressed with the fact that these people were getting along in heavy jobs," says Dr. Thomas Nale, Union Carbide's medical director, "so we began taking another look at jobs for cardiac patients, with the assumption that we probably had been too easy on these people [thinking it had been] for their own good." Cardiac patients who have healed well and are anxious to work now often resume welding and pipefitting jobs as well as ironworking and rigging, and Dr. Nale notes that the results so far have been excellent.

Dr. James Sterner, medical director for Eastman Kodak, says that about 95 percent of their people who are able to work after a heart attack are now brought back to their old jobs. "This is a remarkable change in our attitude. And it came about because cardiac patients who did go back to their old jobs performed better than we ever thought they could."

The mental benefits of allowing a heart patient to work also are important. "In close to half of the cases we handle, we rate the emotional impact of the illness on the patient as more important than the organic disease itself," states Dr. Hellerstein. "We're increasingly convinced that the benefits of returning to work, such as satisfaction, restoration of self-respect, and relief from financial worry, outweigh the stress itself." Instead of throwing heart patients on the scrap heap, industry is beginning to put their skills and knowledge back to work, to the benefit of all concerned. When we consider that our nation loses over $2.5 billion annually when industrial workers who have had heart attacks are not allowed to return to work, it becomes obvious that we have been wasting a vital resource.

If you have had an encounter with heart disease, as millions do each year, talk to your body. It will listen. Tell it this is not the final chapter but the opening of a new life that could be even healthier and happier than before. Prominent cardiologists and industrial leaders will support you in your adoption of this attitude. As Dr. Harvey Wolinsky of the Mount Sinai Hospital and Medical Center states, "Large numbers of Americans have taken responsibility for their health and have in a short time achieved major, stunning relief from an epidemic disease that had for decades been an increasing scourge."

This book, *The Love-Your-Heart Guide for the 1990s*, provides current information from all over the world to help you begin to make changes in your life to protect your heart. There is a lot that we know now that you can and should do to decrease the likelihood of having a coronary attack, as well as a recurrent attack. You can stop smoking. You can choose to eat a healthy diet, and you can take time to exercise and engage in other activities to alleviate the stress in your life.

As a public health educator and life insurance executive, I have seen too much needless loss of life. Don't be among the millions of men and women who will die of heart disease this year. I hope you will use your new knowledge to protect your heart. To quote John Donne, "Any man's death diminishes me because I am involved in mankind."

Notes

CHAPTER 1

Page 1. **Last year almost a million men and women:** National Heart, Lung, and Blood Institute, *Fact Book for 1979* (Washington, D.C.: National Institutes of Health, no. 80-1674), 25.

Page 1. **A life is taken every 32 seconds:** American Heart Association, *1990 Heart and Stroke Facts* (1990): 1.

Page 3. **In the 1950s a British Research Council study:** J. N. Morris, "Coronary Heart Disease and Physical Activity of Work: Evidence of a National Necropsy Survey," *British Medical Journal* 2 (1958): 1485-96.

Page 3. **Dr. Morris's more recent studies:** J. N. Morris, M. G. Everett et al., "Vigorous Exercise in Leisure Time," *Lancet* 2 (1980): 1207-10.

Page 4. **London bus drivers who sat down:** J. N. Morris, A. Kagan, D. C. Pattison et al., "Incidence and Prediction of Ischemic Heart Disease in London Busmen," *Lancet* 2 (1966): 553-59.

Page 4. **Israeli study of 9,000:** D. Brunner and B. Manelis, "Myocardial Infarction Among Members of Communal Settlements in Israel," *Lancet* 2 (1960): 1049.

Page 4. **United States Centers for Disease Control:** "Inactivity: New Health Risk," *Vogue*, October 1987.

Page 4. **today have high blood pressure:** Henry Black and John Seraro, *Anti-Hypertensive Treatment Consultant* (January 1989): 88.

Page 5. **two-thirds of the necessary nutrients:** U.S. Department of Agriculture, *Study of 1955-1964* (Washington, D.C.: U.S. Department of Agriculture).

Page 5. **a later study by the same group:** United States Department of Health, Education, and Welfare, *Highlights: Ten State Nutrition Survey: 1960-1970* (Washington, D.C.: Department of Health, Education, and Welfare, no. HSM 72-8134).

Page 5. **relationship between diet and heart disease**: K. R. Norum, "Some Present Concepts Concerning Diet and Prevention of Coronary Heart Disease," *Nutrition and Metabolism* 22 (1978): 1-7.

Page 5. **most Americans were still ignoring diet**: Blossom H. Patterson and Gladys Block, "Food Choices: Cancer Guidelines," *American Journal of Public Health* 78, no. 3 (March 1988): 282.

Page 5. **more determined to keep weight down**: quotes from Drs. Herman and Van Sittalie obtained from personal interview with Mrs. Phillip Gillon, April 1976.

Page 5. **more Americans are more overweight**: Gordon Bakoulis, "Where There Is Smoke," *Health Care Digest*, July 1988, 18.

Page 6. **sugar may be just as injurious**: J. Yudkin, *Sweet and Dangerous* (New York: Bantam, 1972).

Page 6. **390,000 heart disease-related**: Centers for Disease Control, *Morbidity and Mortality Weekly Report* 38, no. S-2, 24 March 1989.

Page 6. **smoke affects the heart**: Gordon Bakoulis, "Where There Is Smoke," *Health Care Digest*, July 1988, 18.

Page 7. **can raise blood pressure**: Marvin Moser, High Blood Pressure Information Center, *High Blood Pressure: What You Can Do About It*, publication 120, 80.

Page 7. **How stress affects each individual**: M. Friedman and R. H. Rosenman, *Type A Behavior and Your Heart* (New York: Alfred A. Knopf, 1974).

Page 7. **personality type may not be as important**: David R. Ragland and Richard J. Brand, "Type A Behavior and Mortality from Coronary Heart Disease," *New England Journal of Medicine*, (14 January 1988): 318.

Page 8. **many had the same risk factors**: California Teacher's Association publication, 16 October 1973.

Page 8. **Atherosclerosis and coronary heart disease**: R. G. Voller, Jr. and W. B. Strong, "Is Atherosclerosis a Pediatric Problem?" *American Heart Journal*, 101, no. 6 (1981): 815-36.

Page 8. **evidence of hardening of the coronary arteries**: W. F. Enos, R. H. Holmes, and J. Beyer, "Coronary Disease among United States Soldiers Killed in Action in Korea: Preliminary Report," *Journal of the American Medical Association* 152 (1953): 1090-93.

Page 9. **they would have been prime candidates**: J. J. McNamara, M. A. Molot, J. F. Stremple et al., "Coronary Artery Disease in Combat Casualties in Vietnam," *Journal of the American Medical Association* 216 (1971): 1185-87.

Page 9. **A study of more than 200 pilots**: W. M. Glantz, "Coronary Artery Disease as a Factor in Aircraft Fatalities," *Journal of Aviation Medicine* February 1959.

Page 9. **failed to find a clean artery**: Curtis Mitchell, "New Cure For Sick Hearts," *True*, 1962.

Page 9. **middle age now begins**: Ibid.

Page 9. **the question is not who has atherosclerosis**: National Research Council publication 338, 1954.

Page 10. **3,106 healthy men**: N. C. Ekelund, "Physical Fitness Level Predicts Risk of Heart Attack Death," *Cardiovascular Research Report*, Spring 1987.

Page 10. **estrogen replacement therapy**: Betty Weider, "Mysteries of the Female Heart," *Shape*, February 1990, 18.

CHAPTER 2

Page 14. **men who do not exercise have twice as many heart attacks**: J. Naughton and J. Bruhn, "Emotional Stress, Physical Activity and Ischemic Heart Disease," *Disease-a-Month*, July 1980, 1–34.

Page 14. **increased exercise can definitely help**: S. M. Fox III, J. P. Naughton, and W. L. Haskell, "Physical Activity and the Prevention of Coronary Disease," *Annals of Clinical Research* 3 (1971): 404–32.

Page 14. **"Instead of concentration on cures"**: Dr. Joan Ullyot, *Women's Running* (Mountain View, CA: World Publications, 1976).

Page 15. **what gave Demar**: J. H. Currens and P. D. White, "Half a Century of Running," *New England Journal of Medicine* 265 (1961): 988.

Page 15. **all purpose risk reducer**: Peter Wood, *Run to Health* (New York: Charter Books, 1980).

Pages 15–16. **"Real physical exercise erases mental fatigue"**: K. H. Cooper, *The New Aerobics* (New York: Bantam Books, 1970).

Page 16. **exercise helps alleviate nervous tension**: T. K. Cureton, "Improvement of Psychological States by Means of Exercise-Fitness Programs," *Association for Physical and Mental Rehabilitation Journal* 17 (1963): 14–17.

Page 16. **electrical activity in the muscles**: H. A. DeVries, "Immediate and Long Term Effects of Exercise upon Resting Muscle Action Potential Level 5," *Sports Medicine* 8 (1968): 1–11.

Page 16. **a mere two floors of stairs**: *American Journal of Psychiatry*, December 1960.

Page 17. **supplement the blood supply**: Wildor Holmann, interview conducted at the 16th annual World Congress for Sports Medicine, 12 June 1966, Hanover, Germany.

Page 18. **at least two additional years**: As cited in Ann C. Roark, "Fitness Past 40," *Good Health Magazine*, 8 October 1989, 46.

Page 18. **"all the answers we need"**: Jane Brody, "Exercise Is the Fountain of Youth," *New York Times*, 10 June 1986.

Page 19. **"fountain of youth"**: *LA Times Magazine*, 8 October 1989, 46–54.

Page 19. **prescribe exercise:** Ibid.

Page 19. **doubled the life span:** "Prime Time," a newsletter published by Sutter Resource Communication, Sacramento, CA, Winter 1989.

Page 20. **"heart like the quarterback":** John Davis Cantwell, *Stay Young at Heart* (Chicago: Nelson Hall, 1975), 30.

Page 21. **within your training range:** L. Zohman, "Run for Your Life," a pamphlet issued by the Connecticut Mutual Life Insurance Co., Hartford, 1979.

Page 25. **most benefit in the shortest time:** K. H. Cooper, *The New Aerobics*, (New York: Bantam Books, 1970), 13.

Page 26. **marathoners are not increasing:** Harley Hartung, *Psychology Today*, February 1979, 7.

Page 28. **improve cardiovascular function:** "Swimming Benefit Confirmed for Adults" *Physician and Sports Medicine* 15, no. 7, July 1987, 51–54.

Page 29. **booked eight hours a day:** D. Kullano, *Newsweek*, 14 October 1985.

Page 29. **Dr. Paul Hutinger:** Jane Brody, "Exercise Is the Fountain of Youth," *New York Times*, 10 June 1986.

Page 29. **Dr. Herbert DeVries:** Ibid.

Page 29. **Dr. Clifford Graves:** Ibid.

Page 30. **"don't have the continual pounding":** Dr. Jack Wilmore, from a talk given in Davis, CA, 1980.

Page 31. **"more likely to stick with it":** Jeffrey Tanji, "Exercise—Prescription for Health," *Consultant* 28 (June 1988): 57–63.

Page 32. **control hypertension and discourage:** James M. Rippe, Ann Ward, John Porcari, Patty S. Freedson, "Walking for Health and Fitness," *Journal of the American Medical Association* 2, no. 59 (1988): 2720–24.

Page 33. **low-intensity exercise:** "Can Walking Make You as Fit as Running?" *Running and Fitness* 8, no. 1, January 1990.

Page 34. **men who climbed fewer:** *Lancet* 17 February 1953.

Page 34. **burning 2,000 calories a week:** Michael Yessis, "Up to Fitness," *Shape*, November 1989, 101–102.

Page 35. **maximal oxygen uptake:** L. Zohman, "Run for Your Life," a pamphlet issued by the Connecticut Mutual Life Insurance Co., Hartford, 1979.

Page 36. **showed no significant increase:** T. M. Pollock, "How Much Exercise Is Enough?" *The Physician and Sports Medicine*, June 1978.

Page 36. **thick hearts found in weight lifters:** "The Athlete's Heart: Texas Researchers Report Study Comparing Weight Lifters with Distance Runners," *Cardiovascular Research Report* 8 (Spring 1983).

Page 36. **young people too:** *Journal of the American Medical Association* 260, no. 23 (1988): 3441–45.

Page 36. **steroids increase the overall cholesterol level**: William E. Buckley et al., "Estimated Prevalence of Anabolic Steroid Use Among Male High School Seniors" *Wake Forest University News*, 26 January 1990.

Page 38. **Treadmills are ideal**: Bob Goldman, "Buy the Best— Shape's Guide to Home Gym Equipment," *Shape* (December, 1989): 96–99.

Page 38. **which causes the spine to move**: Valerie De Benedette, "Stair Machines: the Truth About This Fitness Fad," *The Physician and Sports Medicine* 18, No. 6 (June 1990): 131–34.

Page 42. **17,000 Harvard alumni**: R. S. Paffenbarger, Jr., "Physical Activity as an Index of Heart Attack Rise in College Alumni," *American Journal of Epidemiology* 108 (September 1978): 161–75.

Page 44. **Leaves doubles out**: Deborah Franklin and Lisa Davis, [11]Double Your Pleasure, but Not Fitness," *Hippocrates*, November/December 1987, 11.

Page 49. **Physical fitness experts**: W. Drygas and A. Jealer, *International Journal of Sports Medicine* 4 (9 August 1988): 275–78.

Page 49. **"I elect to exercise now"**: P.O. Astrand, presentation at the national Convention of the American Association of Health, Physical Education and Recreation, April 1970, Seattle, Washington.

CHAPTER 3

Page 51. **Surgeon General's Report**: *Surgeon General's Report on Nutrition and Health* (Washington, D.C.: U.S. Government Printing Office, 1988).

Page 51. **Framingham study**: T. R. Dawber, W. B. Kannel et al., "Some Factors Associated with the Development of Coronary Heart Disease: 6-Year Follow-Up Experiment in the Framingham Study," *American Journal of Public Health* 49 (1959): 1249–1356.

Page 51. **correlation of high serum cholesterol**: J. E. Watson, "Diet, Cholesterol and Coronary Heart Disease," *Cardiovascular News* 24, no. 6 (November–December 1988): 44–53; A. R. Walker and H. H. Vorster, "Coronary Heart Disease Avoidance—the Dilemma," *South Africa Medical Journal* 10 (November 1974): 482–84; M. F. Oliver, "Diet and Coronary Risk in Men and Women," *Lancet* 1, no. 8637 (11 March 1989): 564.

Page 52. **people who greatly reduce their cholesterol**: D. H. Blankenhorn, "Prevention or Reversal of Arteriosclerosis: Review of Current Evidence," *American Journal of Cardiology* 62, no. 16 (2 May 1989): 3814–4111.

Page 55. **A high serum triglyceride level**: "High Triglyceride Level Gains Importance as CAD Risk Factor," *Medical World News*, 8 February 1988, 17.

Page 55. **"Milking" the finger**: Stanley Gershoff, "But Is Your Cholesterol Level What They Say It Is?" *Tufts University Diet and Nutrition Letter* 6, no. 12 (February 1989): 7.

Page 62. **Dr. Kannel who directed**: Bray G. A., Gray D.S., Obesity Part I Pathogenesis *Western Journal of Medicine* (October 1988) 149; 429-441.

Page 62. **most important factor was fat**: Cited in Carol Lewis, *Shape*.

Page 62. **overweight were more than three times**: Joann E. Manson et al., "A Prospective Study of Obesity and Risk of Coronary Heart Disease in Women," *New England Journal of Medicine* 322, no. 13 (24 March 1990): 882-89.

Page 63. **diet produced many of the concomitants**: J. Yudkin, *Sweet and Dangerous* (New York: Bantam Books, 1972).

Page 63. **A. M. Cohen of Jerusalem**: A. M. Cohen, S. Bavly, and R. Pusnanski, "Change of Diet of Yemenite Jews in Relation to Diabetes and Ischemic Heart Disease," *Lancet* 2 (1961): 1399-1401.

Page 63. **Eskimos who lived near white settlements**: Otto Schaeffer, "When the Eskimo Comes to Town," *Nutrition Today*, November/December 1971, 8-16.

Page 63. **sugar (especially in ice cream)**: M. Friedman and R. H. Rosenman, *Type A Behavior and Your Heart* (New York: Alfred A. Knopf, 1974).

Page 63. **Many other foods**: "Too Much Sugar," *Consumer Union*, March 1978.

Page 65. **rate is higher in Hawaii**: T. L. Robertson, H. Ksto, J. Gordan et al., "Epidemiologic Studies of Coronary Heart Disease and Stroke in Japanese Men Living in Japan, Hawaii, and California: Coronary Heart Disease Risk Factors in Japan and Hawaii," *American Journal of Cardiology* 39 (1977): 244-49.

Page 65. **A study of about 3,300 Chinese**: Whitemore, A. F.; W. V. Williams A. H. et al., "Diet, Physical Activity and Colorectal Cancer Among Chinese in North America and China," *Journal of the National Cancer Institute* 82, Number 11 (June 6, 1990): 915-26.

Page 66. **The oil found in fish can greatly lower**: W. S. Harris and W. E. Connor, "The Effects of Salmon Oil upon Plasma Lipids, Lipoproteins and Triglyceride Clearance," *Transactions of the Association of American Physicians* 93 (1980) 148-155.

Page 66. **fish oil supplements**: Stanley Gershoff, "Paddle the Other Way," *Tufts University Diet and Nutrition Letter* 7, no. 12 (February 1990).

Page 67. **others question this substitution**: K. A. Oster, "Duplicity in a Committee Report on Diet and Coronary Heart Disease," *American Heart Journal* 99 (1980): 409-12; J. D. Weihrauch, C. A. Brignoli, J. B. Reeves et al., "Fatty Acid Composition of Margarine, Processed Fats, and Oils: A New Complication of Data for Tables of Food Composition," *Food Technology* 31 (1980): 80-85.

Page 67. **now cheeses in supermarkets:** "Say Cheese with Discretion," *Tufts University Diet and Nutrition Letter* 6, no. 10 (December 1988): 7.

Page 68. **vegetable and fruit group:** M. G. Hardinge, A. C. Chambers, H. Crooks et al., "Nutritional Studies of Vegetarians, III. Dietary Levels of Fiber," *American Journal of Clinical Nutrition* 6 (1958): 523.

Page 68. **generous amounts of pectin:** A. G. Shaper and K. W. Jones, "Serum Cholesterol, Diet and Coronary Heart Disease in Africans and Asians in Uganda," *Lancet* (1959): 34.

Page 68. **skins of many fruits:** G. H. Palmer and D. G. Dixon, "Effect of Pectin Dose on Serum Cholesterol Levels," *American Journal of Clinical Nutrition* 18 (1966): 437.

Page 68. **a vegetarian diet:** P. M. Kris-Etherton, Debra Krummel, Darlene Dreon et al., "The Effect of Diet on Plasma Lipids, Lipoproteins, and Coronary Heart Disease," *Journal of the American Dietetic Association* 88, no. 11 (November 1988): 1373–4000.

Page 69. **those who ate large amounts of garlic:** A. K. Bordia, M. K. Josji et al., "Effect of Essential Oil of Garlic on Serum Fibrinolytic Activity in Patients with Coronary Artery Disease," *Atherosclerosis* 128 (1977): 155–59.

Page 69. **garlic distinctly inhibited:** A. K. Bordia, S. K. Verma A. K. Vyas et al., "Effect of Essential Oil of Onion and Garlic on Experimental Atherosclerosis in Rabbits," *Atherosclerosis* 26 (1977): 379–86.

Page 69. **vitamin C, which can lower:** E. Ginter, "Vitamin C Lowers Serum Cholesterol," *Science* 16 (February 1973): 66.

Page 76. **"by-products of a maladaptive diet":** J. H. O'Keefe, Jr. and J. C. O'Keefe, "Ventricular Arrhythmas Complicating Weight Reduction Therapy in a Patient with a Privileged QT Interval," *Postgraduate Medicine* 6 (May 1985): 243–50.

CHAPTER 4

Page 78. **eighth graders have elevated:** David E. Fixler et al., "Hypertension Screening in Schools: Results of the Dallas Study," *Pediatrics* 63 (1979): 32–36.

Page 78. **high blood pressure is increasing:** M. D. Sweet and M. J. Dillon, "Hypertension in Children," *British Medical Journal* 299 (19 August 1989): 469–71.

Page 79. **"A University of Michigan study":** T. Irwin, "Watch Your Blood Pressure," Public Affairs Pamphlet no. 483 (New York: Public Affairs Committee, 1975), 8.

Page 79. **"dominant, assertive and decisive":** Ibid.

Page 80. **suppressed hostility:** J. Dinsdale, "Anger and Blood Pressure," *Drug Therapy* June 1989, 105.

Page 80. **San Francisco city bus drivers**: American Heart Association, "Are Bus Drivers Driven to High Blood Pressure?" *Cardiovascular Research Report* Spring/Summer 1986, 4.

Page 82. **stroke hits the right side**: *Health Scene*, Summer 1987.

Page 84. **undetected high blood pressure**: W. B. Kannel, T. Gordon, and M. J. Schwartz, "Systolic Versus Diastolic Blood Pressure and Risk of Coronary Heart Disease: The Framingham Study," *American Journal of Cardiology* 27 (1971): 335.

Page 86. **both numbers are important**: T. Dawber, *The Framingham Study: The Epidemiology of Atherosclerotic Disease* (Cambridge, MA: Harvard University Press, 1980), 80.

Page 87. **Joint National Committee**: Cited in "What Is High Blood Pressure?" *Sacramento Bee*, 14 January 1977.

Page 87. **remarkably free from hypertension**: W. J. Oliver, E. L. Cohen, and J. V. Neel, "Blood Pressure, Sodium Intake, and Sodium-Related Hormones in the Yanomamo Indians in a 'No Salt' Culture," *Circulation* 52 (1975): 46–51.

Page 87. **high incidence of hypertension**: T. Sata et al., "The Relation between Gastric Cancer Mortality Rate and Salted Food Intake in Several Places in Japan," *Bulletin of the Institute of Public Health (Japan)* (1959): 191–95.

Page 92. **"the Chinese restaurant syndrome"**: H. H. Schaumberg, R. Byck, R. Gertsl et al., "Monosodium Glutamate: Its Pharmacology and Role in the Chinese Restaurant Syndrome," *Science* 163 (1969): 32–36.

Page 94. **"protection from the potassium"**: L. Tobian, "How to Deal with Essential Hypertension Determinates of Health: What Doctors Can Do to Decrease the Risk of Coronary Artery Disease," talk given at the Coronary Artery Disease Symposium at the University of Arizona College of Medicine, 19 March 1981.

Page 94. **bachelors die earlier**: Associated Press, Annual Meeting, American Heart Association, New Orleans.

Page 95. **calcium supplementation may lower**: Richard D. Bukoski and David A. McCarron, "Calcium Supplementation May Lower Hypertension," *Drug Therapy*, November 1986, 73.

Page 96. **switched to decaffeinated coffee**: Lawrence E. Lamb, "Decaffeinated Coffee and Bad Cholesterol," *Health Letter* 35, no. 1, 12 January 1990.

Page 96. **suppressed hostility**: J. Dinsdale, "Anger and Blood Pressure," *Drug Therapy*, June 1989, 105.

Page 97. **blood pressure was highest**: Cited in a talk by Walter Schafer at California State University, 1978.

Page 97. **excellent physical shape**: K. Cooper, M. L. Pollock, R. P. Martin et al., "Physical Fitness Levels in Selected Coronary Heart Disease Risk Factors and Physical Fitness in Healthy Women," *Circulation* 67 (1983): 977.

Page 98. **exercise lowered participants' blood pressures:** "Heartbeat," *Cooking Light*, May/June 1989, 18.

Page 98. **14,988 male Harvard alumni:** Paffenbarger et al., "Physical Activity, All-Cause Mortality and Longevity of College Alumni," *New England Journal of Medicine* 314, no. 10 (6 March 1986): 605-13.

Page 98. **light jogging, walking, or swimming:** John L. Boyer and Fred W. Kasch, "Exercise Therapy in Hypertensive Men," *Journal of the American Medical Association* 211 (1970): 1668-71.

Page 100. **cost of medication:** E. J. Roccella, "Cost of Hypertension Medications: Is It a Barrier to Hypertension Control?" *Geriatrics* 44 (October 1989, supp. B): 49-55.

CHAPTER 5

Page 103. **"At any age, smoking increases":** William Bennett, "The Cigarette Century," *Science* 80 (September/October 1980): 43.

Page 103. **association between cigarette smoking:** C. C. Seltzer, "Smoking and Coronary Heart Disease: What Are We to Believe?" *American Heart Journal* 100 (September 1980): 276-80.

Page 104. **women are more prone:** "Smoking Clouds Women's Life Span Outlook," *California Association of Life Underwriters Newsletter*, January 1977.

Page 104. **affects their fertility:** "Cigarette Smoke and Women," *Mayo Clinic Health Letter*, April 1987.

Page 105. **include a greater risk:** Ibid.

Page 106. **yearly radiation dose:** Lowell Ponte, "Radioactivity: the New-Found Danger in Cigarettes," *Reader's Digest*, March 1986.

Page 107. **11 percent decrease:** J. A. Morrison et al., "Cigarette Smoking, Alcohol Intake, and Oral Contraceptives: Relationship to Lipids and Lipoproteins in Adolescent School Children," *Metabolism* 11 (November 1979): 1166-70.

Page 108. **alter levels of sex hormones:** *American Health*, June 1989.

Page 108. **association of smoking with carotid atherosclerosis:** American Heart Association National Center news release, 10 July 1989.

Page 109. **National Academy of Science:** "Passive Smoking and Lung Cancer—What Is the Risk?" *American Review of Respiratory Disease* 133 (1986): 1-3.

Page 110. **sitting near cigarette smokers:** W. Aronow, "Effect of Passive Smoking on Angina Pectoris," *New England Journal of Medicine* 299 (July 1978): 21-24.

Page 110. **incidence of respiratory illnesses**: "Passive Smoking: Effects on Children," *California Pediatrician*, Spring 1988.

Page 111. **wives of never-smokers**: Lawrence E. Lamb, *The Health Letter* 29, no. 6, (March 1987): 4.

Page 111. **other people's tobacco smoke**: *The Health Consequences of Involuntary Smoking*, report of the U.S. Surgeon General (Rockville, MD: Office on Smoking and Health, 1988).

Page 113. **two years after quitting**: Harvey Wolinsky, "Taking Heart," *The Sciences*, February 1981, 7.

Page 114. **nicotine jolts**: William Bennett, "The Cigarette Century," *Science* 80 (September/October 1980): 43.

Page 114. **"cold turkey"**: G. D. Friedman and A. B. Siegelaub, "Changes After Quitting Cigarette Smoking," *Circulation* 61 (1980): 716-23.

Page 115. **lead to some weight gain**: Hiroshi Shimokata, Denis C. Muller, and Reuben Andres, "Studies in the Distribution of Body Fat: Effects of Cigarette Smoking," *Journal of the American Medical Association* 261, no. 8 (24 February 1989): 1169.

Page 115. **increase in waist-hip ratios**: Ibid.

Page 115. **a large number of young people**: Ibid.

Page 115. **toxic and no alternative**: J. R. Palmer, L. Rosenberg, and S. Shapiro, "Low Yield Cigarettes and the Risk of Non-Fatal Myocardial Infarction in Women," *New England Journal of Medicine* 320, no. 24 (15 June 1989): 1569-73.

Page 118. **significant amount of carbon monoxide**: University of California, Berkeley, *Wellness Letter*, March 1979.

CHAPTER 6

Page 125. **change in an individual's life pattern**: "Stress: Can We Cope?" *Time*, 6 June 1983.

Page 125. **Holmes-Rahe scale**: T. Holmes and N. Masada, "Psychosomatic Syndrome," *Psychology Today*, April 1972.

Page 126. **tallying up the life-stress points**: R. H. Rahe, "Life Change Events and Relative Stress," *American Journal of Psychiatry* (1973): 130-222.

Page 126. **"may well be the same"**: Hans Selye, *The Stress of Life* (New York: McGraw-Hill, 1976).

Page 128. **person's appraisal of the situation**: Richard S. Lazarus, "Little Hassles Can Be Hazardous to Health," *Psychology Today*, July 1981, 58-62.

Page 128. **"live in a world of uncertainties"**: Herbert Benson, *The Relaxation Response* (New York: William Morrow, 1975): 18.

Page 129. **not one had a heart attack**: R. Rosenman et al., "Coronary Heart Disease in the Western Collaborative Group Study: Final Follow-Up Experience of 8½ Years," *Journal of the American Medical Association* 223 (August 1975): 872-77.

Page 129. **ratio of Type A's to Type B's:** "Altering Type A Behavior: Up for Debate" *Medical World News,* 14 April 1986.

Page 132. **Richard Nixon:** Richard Nixon, "I Could See No Reason to Live," *Time,* 2 April 1990, 35.

Page 132. **Type C's are completely opposite:** Gary Kamiya, "The Cancer Personality," *Hippocrates,* November/December 1989: 92–93.

Page 133. **clusters of personality traits:** M. Freidman and R. H. Rosenman, *Type A Behavior and Your Heart* (New York: Alfred A. Knopf, 1974); Ernst and Roberts, *Journal of Psychological Type* 15 (1988): 3.

Page 133. **higher heart rate:** Walt Schafer, *Stress, Distress and Growth* (Davis, CA: International Dialogue Press, 1978): 83.

Page 134. **brain activity alone:** "Scientists: Stress Triggers Most Killer Heart Attacks," *Sacramento Bee,* 9 November 1978, 11.

Page 134. **higher hostility scores:** Jerry Bishop, "Hostility, Distrust May Put Type A's at Coronary Risk," *Wall Street Journal* January 17, 1989: B1.

Page 135. **releases fatty acids:** P. Oglesby, "Myocardial Infarction and Sudden Death," *Hospital Practice* 6 (1971): 91–103.

Page 135. **A lot of people:** P. Oglesby. "Myocardial Infarction and Sudden Death," *Hospital Practice* 6 (1971): 91–103.

Page 137. **high job control and low psychological demands:** "Heart Disease and Job Stress: Your Work Can Do You In," *Health Scene* (Sutter Hospital, Sacramento), Winter 1988.

Page 138. **This realization is not new.** H. Russek, "Emotional Stress and Coronary Heart Disease in American Physicians, Dentists, and Lawyers," *American Journal of Medical Science,* 243 (1962): 716–26.

Page 139. **top executives of both:** "Longevity of Corporate Executives," *Metropolitan Life Statistical Bulletin,* February 1974, 13–14.

Page 140. **270,000 employees:** L. E. Hinkle, Jr. et al., "Occupation, Education, and Coronary Heart Disease," *Science* 161 (1968): 238–46.

Page 140. **"nervous system improves its capacity":** From a talk given by Ralph W. Gerard at a symposium at the University of California Medical Center, San Francisco, 1963.

Page 141. **higher rate of sudden death:** R. S. Eliot, *Stress and the Major Cardiovascular Disorders* (New York: Future Publishing, 1979), 10.

Page 141. **Similarly, Friedman and Rosenman.** M. Friedman, R. H. Rosenman and V. Carroll, "Change in the Serum Cholesterol and Blood Clotting Time in Men Subjected to Cycstic Variation," *U.S. Occupational Stress Circulation* 1958, 18: 852–61.

Page 141. **American Psychological Association's meeting:** "Stress Takes Its Toll on Housewives," *Sacramento Union,* 1 September 1985.

Page 142. **At the age of 44.** Dennis L. Breo, "Is it Worth Dying

For?" *American Medical News* 15 May 1984: 24-6.

Page 142. **$5,152 in medical costs:** From a meeting with Equitable Life Insurance executives, 1985.

Page 147. **pets have a tranquilizing effect:** A. H. Katcher, E. Friedman, A. M. Beck, et al., "Looking, Talking, and Blood Pressure: The Physiological Consequences of Interaction with the Living Environment," in A. H. Katcher and A. M. Beck (eds.), *New Perspectives in Our Lives with Companion Animals* (Philadelphia: University of Pennsylvania Press, 1983): 351-59.

Page 147. **Dr. William Fry:** cited in Jane Brody, "Personal Health," *New York Times,* 7 April 1988.

Page 148. **Dr. Marvin Eitterring:** Ibid.

CHAPTER 7

Page 151. **muscular effort with fewer heartbeats:** H. K. Hellerstein, "Exercise Therapy in Coronary Disease," *Bulletin of the New York Academy of Medicine* 44 (1968): 1028-47.

Page 151. **program of acute and ambulatory:** N. K. Wenger and H. K. Hellerstein (eds.), *Rehabilitation of the Coronary Patient* (New York: John Wiley & Sons, 1978).

Page 156. **follow Dr. Kavanagh's instructions:** T. Kavanagh, "Keep Your Heart in Shape: Run for Your Life," *Round Table Magazine,* September 1976.

Page 156. **The Japanese are most interested:** T. Kavanagh, "Cardiac Rehabilitation and Return to Work," *Sanylka Oaigaku Zasshi* 11 (20 March 1989) (Supp. 1): 49-62.

Page 157. **heart patients and others can derive:** Ezra A. Amsterdam, Lawrence J. Laslett, Rudolph H. Dressendorfer, and Dean T. Mason, "Exercise Training in Coronary Heart Disease: Is There a Cardiac Effect?" *American Heart Journal 101* (June 1981): 870-3.

Page 157. **"after acute myocardial infarction":** E. A. Amsterdam, J. H. Wilmore, and A. N. Dermaria, *Exercise in Cardiovascular Health and Disease* (New York: New York Medical Books, 1978).

Page 157. **save approximately 13,000 lives:** G. T. O'Connor, R. Collins, et al., "Rehabilitation," *Circulation* 82 (1989): 234-44.

Page 157. **vascular complications:** P. Greenland and J. Chu, "Cardiac Rehabilitation Services and Risk Reduction," *Annals of Internal Medicine* 3, no. 3 (1 August 1989).

Page 158. **adding other treatments:** A. Oberman, "Rehabilitation of Patients with Coronary Artery disease," in E. Braunwald (ed.), *Heart Disease: A Textbook of Cardiovascular Medicine* (Philadelphia: W. B. Saunders, 1988): 1395-1409.

Page 159. **Sex with someone:** Cleveland and Japanese studies cited in *The Medical Forum,* HMS health letter (March 1986): 5-6.

Page 161. **"Americans have taken responsibility":** Harvey Wolinsky, "Taking Heart," *The Sciences* (February 1981).

Index